I dedicate this book to my former self.
This book would not have been possible without you.
Thank you for the memories.

I STRUGGLED WITH OBESITY AND SURVIVED

My Painful Journey

AMON RAO

ABOUT THE AUTHOR

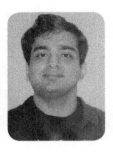

Amon Rao was born in the Fiji Islands in 1984 and obtained his primary education in Fiji and Scotland and secondary education in Melbourne. After completing a master's degree in commerce from Sydney University, he became a software developer and a weight-loss coach. He firmly believed that everybody had the ability to lose weight and obtain their dream body. Amon had experienced obesity by the age of six and struggled with this issue for most of his life. By the time he was twenty-one years old, he weighed 180 kilos. Over a period of five years he indulged in a range of physical activities and dieting to fight this weighty problem. Amon had left a draft of this manuscript a week before his untimely death in 2016.

Published in Australia by Sid Harta Publishers Pty Ltd,
ABN: 46 119 415 842
23 Stirling Crescent, Glen Waverley, Victoria 3150 Australia
Telephone: +61 3 9560 9920, Facsimile: +61 3 9545 1742
E-mail: author@sidharta.com.au

First published in Australia 2017
This edition published 2017
Copyright © Amon Rao 2017
Revised by Cecilia Rao and Dr. D. Rao
Cover design, typesetting: WorkingType (www.workingtype.com.au)

Rao, Amon
I struggled with Obesity and Survived – My Painful Journey
ISBN: 978-1-921362-94-1
pp148

CONTENTS

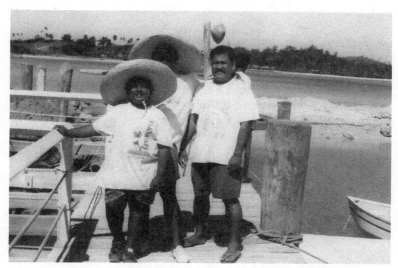

Author (front with hat) at a tourist resort in Fiji (1993)

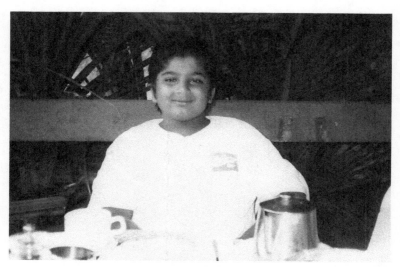

Author (1994)

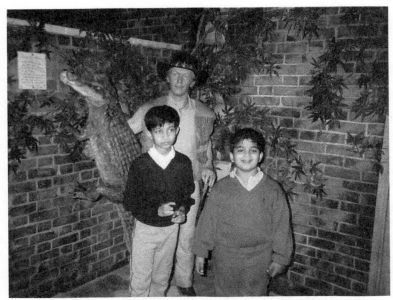

Author (front right) posing in front of the wax of actor Paul Hogan, Madame Tussauds Wax Museum, London (1992)

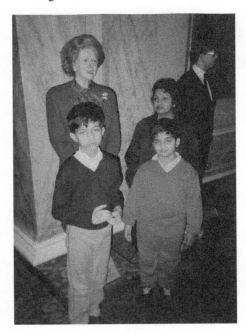

Author (front right) posing in front of the wax of Margaret Thatcher, Madam Tussauds Wax Museum, London, 1992)

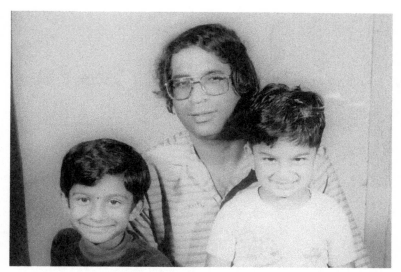

Author (right) posing with dad and brother (1987).

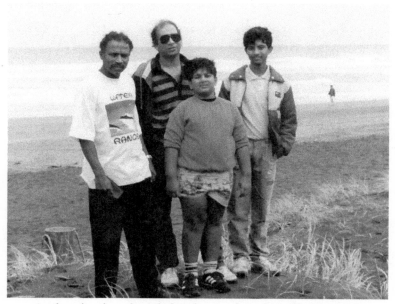

Author (in shorts) with family members (Auckland 1993).

Preface

R ecently our son Amon Rao, aged thirty-two years, died of cardiac arrest while being a patient at Liverpool Hospital. The post mortem report showed that obesity was the primary cause of his death. He had fought this issue over several years and described his experience of his struggle in a moving draft of a book which he had completed just a few weeks before passing away. In this manuscript, Amon described in detail his cruel and humiliating experience at being obese and his rigorous resort to dieting and exercising, which he referred to as my "Journey". Alternatively, he used words such as 'efforts', 'initiatives', 'objectives', 'mission', 'goals', 'endeavour' and 'strategies' to describe his struggle from the beginning to the end to mean the same thing.

Obesity is the world's fastest and alarmingly developing health issue. About 27.5% of Australian children between the ages 5-17 and about two billion people world-wide are obese, according to Leeder (2017). Another study carried out by the Australian researchers and briefly discussed in the Daily Telegraph (Peel: 2017) found that one in five Australian children is overweight prior to schooling, which costs taxpayers $17 million a year. It also reported that the healthcare costs of an obese child under the age of five are $367 higher than a healthy child. Like many other previous research findings, this study also linked obesity to "poor diet" and "lack of exercise."

Doctors, dieticians and other health professionals invariably advise people facing weighty problems to consume foods that contain low calories. Unfortunately, it is not safe to factor in calories only in weight reduction activities, for there are many other

1

factors that have been found to contribute to obesity. Martin (2017), for example, is one such critic of calorie counting:

Excluding waste and sweating, it's true that the calories we take in have to be turned into either energy or weight. So, it ought to be true that taking in less will cut weight. But what usually happens first is that we get hungry (and add back the calories, leaving our weight unchanged) or lethargic (expending less energy so that more of what we take in is directed to maintain our weight. (Sunday-The Sun Herald, Jan 1, 2017:30).

Martin (2017) further states: "It's almost as if our weight wants to be maintained; as if it has a will of its own and manipulates the rest of us to get what it wants. Which is probably what happens." (p. 30). There may be a lot of truth in this observation, for a large percentage of people embarking on weight reduction initiatives quit after a short time because they are not able to tame their recalcitrant bodies which seem to resist change. But those people who defy the instructions of their bodies and continue with their weight reduction strategies seem to complete their Journey and ultimately triumph.

But the study of obesity is not as easy as it sounds. Even scientists up till today have not been able to identify the main cause of obesity. Genetics certainly seem to play a bigger role, as evidenced by the huge bodies carried by many people in some countries in the South Pacific. But in our two families there is not a single person who could be considered obese, except an auntie of ours who at the age of ninety-two years is extremely obese but so far has not shown any evidence of having suffered from a cardiovascular disease.

Our son had stated in his book that at one time he weighed 180kg. But there are thousands of people living in Australia and in other parts of the world who weigh more than 180kg and are surviving. Our son was definitely obese, but he was not the lazy type. He was very active in life and knew the danger of possessing an overweight body. Prior to his death he had satisfactorily completed his Journey. Just a few months before his death, he weighed about 90kg. Sadly, though he had successfully completed his Journey he did not live long to enjoy its aftermath.

What our son had demonstrated is that it is not difficult to overcome obesity as long as a person has the courage, tenacity, and determination to survive. The absence of these characteristics will make the Journey a bit more difficult to complete. Furthermore, a person undertaking the Journey should not expect quick results, like the disappearance of a headache after taking a few tablets of Panadol. Our son had thought that he would be able to shape his body within a few months, but it took him more than two years to get the expected results. Since he lacked patience, I have no doubt that he must have decided to quit his Journey for good on several occasions, but continued on because he expressed to us on a few occasions how beautiful nature was and how he wanted to enjoy being part of it for as long as he could.

Our son was admitted to the hospital on two occasions before his death, due to complications related to Crohn's disease. He was scheduled for release on the day he died. The irony is that he did not die from the disease for which he was admitted to the hospital. We think he had been loading his body with a variety of 'substances' that guaranteed quick weight reduction, which he had obtained online. It seems that these substances interacted toxically with his rigorous exercising and dieting routines, and his body at some stage became so 'overloaded' that his heart could no longer take the extraordinary weight and thus stopped forever.

Please, parents, do something for your overweight child before this 'curse' starts to overwhelm them. We know that it is a common practice for a child to reluctantly convey their personal problems to parents and it is for this reason that you should always look out for negative signals from your child and respond accordingly. You must intervene even if they oppose your 'intrusion' with insults, because the loss of a child is the most painful experience any parent will encounter until death.

Obviously, this story was written by our son to let you readers and sufferers obtain a better understanding of the pain of a person growing up with obesity. We have no doubt that some of you may have already formed an adverse opinion on some of the thoughts our son had expressed. We do not have a quarrel with that, but by just reading this book from the beginning to the end we sincerely believe you will show ample empathy to our son for his miserable suffering.

Cecilia Rao and Dr. D. Rao
Liverpool, Sydney
Australia
11th July 2017

INTRODUCTION

Dear Reader,

I would like to thank you for taking time to read this book. I am confident that it contains a lot of information and guidance needed by you to implement a solid weight loss plan to counter your weight issues.

I have written this narrative for teenagers and adults who are struggling with obesity, and is a useful guide for all other individuals who have struggled with this issue since childhood and have carried this problem into adulthood. Other parents who currently have an overweight kid and require assistance in creating a strategy to address this issue will also find this book very informative.

I know firsthand how limiting it can be growing up and living a life with a body that was abnormally large. I have been there. Hated it. It is definitely not a time I look back upon with fond memories.

In this book, I have written my experiences of being an overweight teenager and transitioning into an adult including the steps I took to turn my life around. This book contains some valuable insights into my excruciating struggle and it also explains various tactics and strategies I utilised to build the mindset needed to blast off the extra weight and fat from my body. If after reading this book you enrol your child for the Journey, I salute you for making this critical decision on behalf of your child. A life without limitation will await your child.

CHAPTER 1

Epidemic Overview

When I was young I remember I often shouted, "When I grow up, I want to be fat." Little did I realise at that time that this slogan would become a reality and become a source of depression, anxiety and monomania later in life.

We are currently experiencing an obesity epidemic globally, and Australia is currently one of the nations leading the way. This country has been recognised as being one of the fattest nations in the world. Statistics provided by the Australia Bureau of Statistics show that 63.4% of Australian adults were overweight or obese in 2014 — 2015. That equates to approximately 11.3 million adults living in the country. Further statistics also indicate that around one in four children aged between 5 — 17 years were overweight or obese in the same years. This equated to approximately 27.4% of children living in Australia. These figures are of huge concern as obesity is known to increase the risk of other major health problems such as type 2 diabetes, coronary heart disease, high blood pressure and cancer, all of which can not only severely impact upon a person's quality of life, but could see them face the prospect of paying enormous medical bills while fighting this problem.

Being overweight can also lead to the development of severe psychological issues such as low self-esteem, negative body image, self-hatred, self-consciousness in the public space and social exclusion. These issues can really distort how such people see themselves and the world. By feeling that they cannot meet society's expectations, they may completely withdraw from society and never give themselves the opportunity to ever be happy.

Obese people also tend to suffer from discrimination in our society, and are usually portrayed as being lazy, greedy and unattractive. They are routinely ostracised and harshly judged. This ensures that they quickly learn that they are inferior compared to their thinner counterparts. The media further makes matters worse by continually ridiculing them on TV shows and movies, and routinely focuses on their negative aspects while rarely showing them in a positive light.

With due respect to obese patients, people in health care see them the very way the community sees them — with disdain and similar to drug addicts, as if they've inflicted obesity on to themselves. These people are bingeing for a reason. Nutritional information and suggestions of smaller meals don't seem to work. Psychologists might diagnose them as suffering from depression, anxiety, or bipolar, and yet they just give them medicine which also promote more weigh-gain.

It is unfortunate that our society still fails to fully understand the physical and psychological problems that overweight people face. They need a lot of courage and effort to live from day to day. Given the lack of consideration shown towards these people, each day for these individuals can be very unfulfilling and disheartening.

On the flipside though, while we can argue that more can be done for overweight people, fault should also be placed on them as they themselves are neglecting their own health. They generally do not like hearing the truth about their weight and instead focus their time and energy on whingeing, blaming, complaining and crying instead of accepting personal responsibility for their health.

Thankfully there are some organisations, support groups and individuals in our community who are trying to make a difference to these people's lives. From raising public awareness about obesity to fighting for healthier foods on our supermarket shelves, these people are our true heroes and we thank them for doing a wonderful work. However, there is a limitation to what these community groups can do to assist these obese group of people.

With no foreseeable solution in sight, obesity rates are expected to continue rising, and it has been forecasted that by 2020 65% of young Australians would be considered overweight.

Growing Up

I have been obese for the most part of my life. I have had the unpleasant 'joy' of being affected by obesity as a child and right into early adulthood. However, I was not born obese, but had reached that level very early in my life. From all the photos that I have of myself as a child, I can conclusively say that I was obese by the age of six. I remember I was about eight years old when my parents took me to a dietician for the very first time, and it was at this age that I was put on my first diet. This was before I even knew what it meant to be healthy. It was at the age of thirteen when I first became self-conscious and embarrassed by the way I looked. This was also the same year I had started going to a mixed school. I had been attending an all-boy's school prior to this. However, I still remember how uncomfortable I felt being in my ugly body at that age, especially now that there were girls around. Every day, I wished I could wake up and be thin. At the age of fifteen, I migrated to Australia with my family. Even though I had made a commitment to lose weight once I arrived here, I found transitioning to my new environment extremely difficult. As a result, I used food as a coping mechanism and found myself piling on weight very quickly. Eventually, I became the fattest guy in my entire school and consequently became severely depressed. One of the first things I learnt early in life was that having a large body in childhood was not easy, nor fun. I had made myself an easy target for ridicule, and found myself regularly being teased by family and friends. I also could not enjoy any family functions without my relatives giving me a lecture on the importance of weight loss. There was a never-ending pressure from their side for me to lose weight, and I was continually expected to meet their unrealistic expectations. However, the worst part of my life as an overweight boy occurred when I started schooling. It was mental and physical torture trying to get through each day at school. My entire life for the most part thus had revolved around my weight and how to lose it. It had been all about dieting, exercising and trying my best to meet society's expectations. While my friends and families had enjoyed socialising, travelling, and dating, among other activities, I generally missed out on these experiences. I always felt that there was something wrong with me. That something was that I was not normal. I had always tried my best to feel accepted, but it was very challenging. I had always felt that losing weight would solve my problems. However, at the age of twenty, I set a new personal weight record. I was tipping the scales at 180 kilograms. It was the lowest point in my life. I was completely lost and did not know which road to follow. Worst of all, my parents had left Australia to work overseas and I should have followed them, but then my teenage life in Australia was irresistible, so I stayed put.

Finding the Root Cause

I was in my late twenties when I finally decided that I would earnestly commit myself to take greater personal responsibility for my health. In the previous years, I had undertaken a few weight management initiatives to address my weight problems, but I was not able to sustain my strategy long enough to see any visible results. I always fell into a relapse within three months. The next time, however, I tried a different approach. Instead of dieting and exercising with the intention and hope of getting a quick result, I tried instead to find the root cause of my problem, and then use the knowledge gained to use the most appropriate strategies at weight reduction.

It had never occurred to me that I had gone through most of my life completely oblivious to the root cause of my weight gain — the real reasons for me being overweight. All I ever heard from others was that I was overweight, and that I needed to go on a diet and exercise to trim my weight. They made it sound very simple. However, no one ever bothered to explain to me the "why" aspect. Instead of asking why I was overweight, I seemed to be too obsessed on controlling the weight gain itself.

As I grew older, I started educating myself on topics related to health, nutrition, exercise and psychology. It was during this time that I stumbled upon a video by Lustig titled Sugar: The Bitter Truth. (http//www.uctv.tv/Shows/Sugar-The-Bitter-Truth-16717).

Sugar is one of the most addictive substances that is currently legally available to the population of this world. Researchers have claimed that sugar is more addictive than heroin, causes great damage to health and is the primary cause of the obesity crisis currently faced by millions of people. I was metamorphosed after watching the Lustig video; I was not the same person anymore. It educated me a lot about my own eating habits and taught me a lot more about my eating problem.

During my formative years, my parents hired a nanny to look after me during the day as both were working full time. The nanny was responsible not only for my daily care but also to feed me properly. This is where I felt the root cause of my obesity had its origin. My nanny was very generous when feeding me with sugar. I remember she put in a lot of sugar in my breakfast. Consequently, it did not take long for me to develop a liking for this ingredient. So, I demanded more sugar in my breakfast when my mother fed me. Because she was not as generous as my nanny, I would not eat unless my mum indulged me with heaps of sugar. At that time, I would have been around three or four years old.

As I grew up and started to face life's challenges, I quickly started consuming sugar as a source of comfort. As my upbringing was not the best, the instant 'high excitement' that came with sugar consumption provided me with the temporary relief that I needed to emotionally cope with myself.

One of the most unfortunate truths during my youthful life was that people in those years had very little knowledge of the deleterious effects of sugar consumption. My friends used to laugh at me when I told them about my addiction to sugar. My parent's attitude was even worse: they saw me just as a person who did not care about health and felt strongly that it was their parental duty to lecture me on a daily basis. Surprisingly, they did not take any concrete steps to hinder my access to the sugar bowl. My parents were also busy dealing with their own problems and might have felt that my addictive behaviour was temporary and would peter out with the passage of time.

My addiction to sugar intensified when I migrated to Australia. Suddenly, I found myself gaining unhindered access not only to sugar but also to products containing a large percentage of sugar. The supermarkets were full of cheap, junk, and sugary food. There was cheap sugar everywhere and I spent years of my useful life feeding my addiction to this product instead of experiencing a normal and balanced life.

The Vicious Cycle of Obesity

Due to my sugar addiction and the subsequent weight gain, life had become very difficult. My ever-increasing weight was affecting me in all areas of my life and I found myself falling many times into a vicious cycle of continuous binge eating and dieting. This continuous cycling caused me a lot of pain and my health was getting damaged.

The diagrams in Figures 1 and 2 outline the two vicious cycles around which I had cycled regularly. To address these serious issues, I felt that I had no choice except to go on dieting. However, since I had taken an unrealistic approach which was not addressing the root cause of my medical problem, I found myself falling into a relapse each time I went on dieting. This meant that as soon as I started to lose weight, I suddenly found myself back to binge eating sugary food. Consequently, my weight increased and my psychological problems intensified. I faced these vicious cycles for many years before I adopted different strategies, which produced much better outcomes.

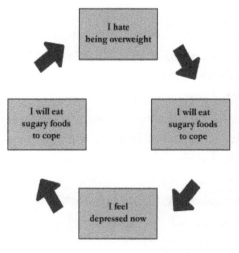

Figure 1: The vicious cycle of obesity

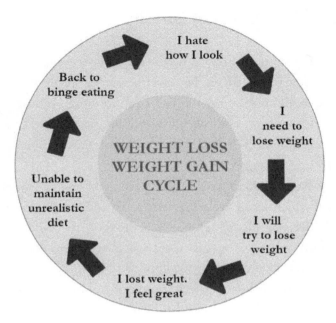

Figure 2: *Weight loss, weight gain cycle*

Taking Action to Change Myself

This isn't the first time I had tried to give up pornography; there had been several unsuccessful attempts over the past years but this time my efforts succeeded completely. Perhaps the most pervasive reason why women ignore their doctors is in their unsubstantiated belief that if they ignore a medical problem, it will just go away. I also held a similar opinion. At the age of twenty-one, my unhealthy eating habits had finally caught up with me. I had been diagnosed with Crohn's disease, an autoimmune disease with no known causes or cure. Consequently, I spent most of my early twenties receiving treatment for this medical condition. I decided to keep this disease a secret and did not reveal anything about it to my family members — not even to my parents. I only disclosed it to my closest friends.

Notwithstanding, my gluttonous habit remained unabated and this exacerbated my medical problem. My craze for sugar became uncontrollable. I went down into a severe depression which caused me to further neglect my health. The medical treatment that I received could not mitigate the problems associated with Crohn's and eventually my bowels perforated. I had to undergo an emergency surgery and woke up post-surgery carrying a colostomy bag. This was one of the toughest moments in my life. I felt suicidal. Eventually I disclosed my medical complications to my family and the rest of my friends. They were not shocked or surprised. It seemed to me as if they had expected something of this nature to eventually happen. "Well he never really looked after his health" and "He never listened to us when we used to give him health advice," they said. Admittedly, there was a modicum of truth in such utterances.

I was also very embarrassed, as wearing a colostomy bag was no fun. I never thought something like this could ever happen to me. I wore the colostomy bag for almost a year. I was now known in the family as the guy with the colostomy bag. However, I was very fortunate that my parents were available to take care of me before and after the reversal of the Crohn's operation.

Furthermore. the night after my first operation however was shocking and traumatising. But I came away from this experience with a keen awareness of the transient nature of our existence. I said to myself that I had to be strong and concluded that if I wanted changes in my life then only I could instigate those changes. Nobody else was going to live my life for me, and not, in any case, the type of life I did not cherish. On my bed, every second, I felt distant from my true desires, avoided the world and was afraid to engage with it.

These seconds became the biggest gift of my life, for the idea of the seeds of change germinated in my mind during those seconds.

While wearing a colostomy bag, I decided that I did not want to be in this state any more. I was tired of being fat and sick. I wanted to enjoy my life. I did not want to continue living in the current state any more. I felt as if I was living in hell. I did not want my parents to feel my agony. They were old now and they had their own health problems. I did not want them to care for me anymore. It was time for me to step up and take appropriate action. It was time for me to take responsibility. It was at this stage that I firmly decided that I must reverse my medical situation.

Finding Success

I have come a long way since making a firm decision to change my lifestyle. I have now overcome my addiction to sugar and my health has improved considerably. I am enjoying my life much more than ever before.

If there is one thing that I have learnt during this transformation, it is that success does not come easily. It took me many years before I gained my present self. It took me years of research, dieting, exercising and trial and error methods to finally find the right combination of strategies to achieve the outcomes that suit my new lifestyle. I intend to sustain these outcomes on a long-term basis.

My biggest challenge during my Journey was to persistently overcome a relapse. While previously spending a considerable amount of time and effort to lose weight, I relapsed many times thereby returning to the ugly point of origin. Fortunately, this outcome was not a total failure. I repeated the steps with added vigour, overcame all obstacles and finally completed my Journey. This was the biggest achievement of my life.

Today, even though my life has completely changed for the better, my Journey has not stopped. My past and current struggles to reduce my weight and remain healthy and strong is a lifelong initiative. It is my long-term goal to become a perfect person and never to go back to my old self.

Tell Me Your Story

Now that you are familiar with my Journey, I would appreciate if you would tell me how do you feel about your weighty problem. I do not know for sure how obesity is affecting your life, but I can guess you will be feeling miserable and carrying a lot of painful memories. Based on my experience, I can assure you that gaining a new and better life is possible after defeating obesity with a reasonable amount of sacrifice and effort.

Before I go any further, I would like to ask you the following questions:

- Do you feel that your weight is holding you back in life?
- Do you hate looking at your body in the mirror?
- Do you feel embarrassed going out in public and feel the need to hide behind clothes?
- Do you hate the fact that one of your biggest weaknesses is to appear in front of others?
- Do you avoid social situations because of your weight?
- Do you hate shopping for clothes?
- Do you feel ignored by the opposite sex?
- Are you sick of waiting till dark before going for a walk?
- Do you hate the fact that you never give yourself a chance?
- Are you sick of people reminding you that you need to lose weight?

◆ Are you dreaming of the day when all these issues do not bother you anymore?

My answers to all the above questions is a big "Yes". You see, being obese just sucks. It really does. Not only is it impossible to live a fulfilling and satisfying life when you are on the wrong end of the scale, but the inconsiderate comments made by many people and the media outlets tend to make you feel that your life is worthless. It takes a lot of courage for a person suffering from obesity to live in the current social environment — to go and face the world. However, I wish you to know that I never imagined that I could lose so much weight and sculpt my body into the shape that I had always dreamed about. I never thought I could ever become strong and muscular. In the beginning, when I regularly looked at myself in the mirror I said to myself that there was no way that I could transform myself from being a fat man into a lean person. This meant that I had declared defeat even before giving myself a chance to succeed. I was very negative. However, the day I seriously decided to take responsibility for my healthy lifestyle and mould my body into a delectable shape, was the day I felt my life changed forever — for good.

If you are overweight and serious about weight reduction, I hope by reading my book from the beginning to the end, you will be in a better position to relate your Journey to the one I have just completed. I sincerely hope I have given you sufficient information and knowledge for you to succeed in losing your weight. Your success in the weight reduction therapy will mean that all the answers to the questions that I had raised previously should carry a big "NO!". This will be the definitive moment when you would be able to shout that you are the master of your own body, and not your weight. It is never too late to start building the body that you always dream of.

To all The Parents of an Overweight Child

Dear Parents,

This chapter has been written for you. If you have a child who is severely overweight or obese, I want you to know that you are failing your role as a parent. I want to be brutally honest with you. You should remember that as a parent, it is your duty to take full responsibility and ownership of your child's health. You must remember that your child is dependent on you for nourishment and that it is your responsibility to provide them with nutritional guidance until they are capable of managing their own diet with a knowledgeable mind.

Please do realise that no child wants to go through their life with an overweight and unbalanced body, especially during the formative years of their life. Obesity generates a nightmarish experience and can leave a child mentally scarred forever. Children who are obese usually end up carrying their weight into adulthood, where they end up experiencing a life full of discrimination, humiliation, prejudice and cultural bias.

As an adult, I hated my parents for neglecting my health and turning a blind eye to my weight. I still cannot understand how they allowed me to go through a miserable life like that. I did not know any better as a child. I did not understand the full consequences of my unhealthy eating until later in life. I was under the impression that my weight would sort itself out as I grew older, and I can only guess that my parents thought the same as well. However, that never happened. My health only became a priority for them once I had fallen sick, but it was too late as the damage had already been done. I wish they had done more when I was younger.

Now, I understand that some parents love their kids too much that they allow them to eat anything they want. For other parents, it could be a cultural issue and a sign of prestige. In fact, there could be a host of other reasons why someone would let their children become overweight. However, also do understand the consequence of your actions.

If you have a child who is overweight, please do note that it is never too late for you to introduce measures to bring his/her weight down. Your intervention may invite a huge tantrum and a sad face from them, because they are missing their favourite junk food. However, do realise that they will be healthier and happier in the future if they possess a sustainable and well-balanced body. They will have better life experiences and opportunities, and most importantly, start their adult years with a good health.

So do your children a favour — give them the opportunity to live up to their normal life span. Make their health your number one priority. They will thank you in the future for your intervention.

Importance of Research and Self-Education

To successfully overcome your weight issues, you will need to get into the habit of continually educating yourself. In my case, important areas of self-education were familiarisation with nutrition, health, exercise, human psychology, medicine and literature on obesity. This preliminary exercise is essential as it will ensure that you are continually updating your knowledge base, and have access to new ideas, approaches and methods that you can implement as part of your weight management plan.

The internet is a great resource for uncovering valuable information. It can play a critical role in your weight-loss Journey. Some of the best ideas that I had added to my weight loss plan had come from online sources. As a result, I had made it a habit to regularly watch health documentaries, visited health-related websites and forums, and paid subscriptions on relevant health channels on social media platforms. By maintaining these habits on a regular basis, I ensured that my knowledge was always current. I also ensured that I kept myself open to new and different ideas, even if they initially sounded absurd. For example, some of the best ideas that had accelerated my weight loss progress had come from online sources and they appeared absolutely ridiculous. It is a good policy not to dismiss any information that comes across you without investigating it thoroughly, as one small action initially discarded could have the potential to negatively transform your life.

Another important skill you should cultivate is to utilise the advanced features of an internet search engine. By applying the advanced options available in the internet, you can carry out filter searches based on phrases, language, region, date and many more. All these efforts will ensure that the information you are presented is relevant to your health requirements, and that all the "fluff" is filtered out. These skills were very useful in facilitating my Journey and I would highly recommend that you acquire these skills as well. Knowledge is power. Take time to acquire it.

Chapter 2

Undertaking Change

It must be understood that to achieve your weight loss goals, you will need to undertake change. This is a mandatory requirement, and if you successfully complete your Journey you will never be the same person again. Success in a weight loss initiative is not possible without change and unless you open yourself up to this change, you will continue to remain overweight. To reduce weight, you need to undergo the inevitable change process to break yourself free from your existing lifestyle, the lifestyle that had given you the current weighty body.

The Change Framework

I recommend you to read Stages of Change Model (Prochaska, J. O; DiClemente and Norcross (1992) (See Figure 3 and Table 1) as part of your change framework. Briefly, this model discusses how change can be brought about to addictive behavior - in my case binge eating. This model consists of 6 stages and will enable you to visualise the different stages that you will cover during your weight-loss Journey. If you are reading this book, it is most likely that you are either in the Pre-Contemplation or the Contemplation stage. You have to carefully understand why this model is important before you begin the implementation phase of your Journey.

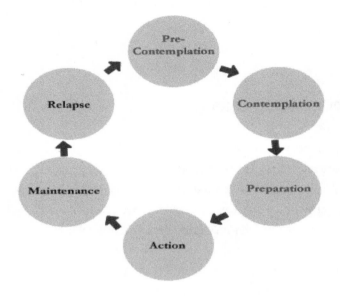

Figure 3: Stages of Change Model (Based on Prochaska, et.al, 1992)

The Change Cycle

When you attempt to implement these strategies of change to yourself, you should count yourself very lucky if you get everything right the first time. However, almost all of you will undoubtedly encounter several minor and major obstacles and setbacks along the way.

As soon as you overcome these obstacles, new ones will present themselves. If you successfully bypass these hurdles head on and keep on moving until to the end, then your ride during your Journey will be a smooth one, if not, then you will be derailed from your path and you will have to restart all over.

STAGE	DEFINITION
Pre-contemplation	In this stage, you are not thinking about losing weight.
Contemplation	In this stage, you are thinking about losing weight.
Preparation	In this stage, you begin making preparations to start your weight loss Journey.
Action	In this stage, you are actively trying to lose weight.
Maintenance	In this stage, you have achieved your weight loss goals and now actively maintaining your new weight results.
Relapse	In this stage, you return to your unhealthy lifestyle.

Table 1: *Explanation of the Stages of Change Model*
(Based on Prochaska, et. al, 1992)

I clearly remember that during my Journey, when I was hovering around the ninety-day mark, I occasionally fell into several relapses. But achieving the ninety-day mark itself in the first attempt boosted my confidence and signaled that my plan was on track, and that attainment of my goals and objectives were within reach. This led me to exercise regularly and eat cleanly, something which I had never done in the past. However, falling into a relapse had made me very miserable and usually led me into depression. But if you show patience, determination and perseverance during your Journey then you should be able to achieve the desired goals in a timely framework.

I acknowledge that it can be hard to overcome a habit that a person has lived with for years, but knowing that your weight problem can be reversed permanently is the trigger that is needed by you to disentangle yourself from this so-called vicious cycle and eventually come out victorious.

Pre-Contemplation

A large percentage of people in the world are not overly concerned about their weight problems. To them, being overweight is not a major health issue.

It has been reported in newspapers and on TV programmes that individuals who are dangerously obese and carry extra weight are unable to leave their bed. They arouse our curiosity as to why on earth they had let their body become such a weighty problem in the first place. Yet, the fact is that this is no longer an unusual occurrence and it means that there is more at work than just individuals eating too much. Obviously, superfluous eating and lack of adequate physical activities may engender weight increase, but the bigger question is why people allow their body to gain weight beyond endurance, which later becomes an impediment to the enjoyment of a balanced lifestyle.

Well, for many of these "big" individuals the negative impacts of their lifestyle have not yet fully manifested themselves. They are under the impression that because they can get up every day and undertake their daily routine without any significant problems, their weight poses no danger to them. Based on this thought, this group of people choose to ignore any information presented to them about the dangers of obesity. For other overweight people, it may be an act of rebelliousness as they do not enjoy being told how they should look. This probably explains why movements such as "Big is beautiful" exist. These people give their situation a political twist and demand acceptance of obesity in the society. Considering that we are currently living in an era of freedom, a large portion of these people feel that they should be accepted for who they are regardless of size. As Robbins (1997: 316-317) says: "A lot of [fat] people know what they should do, but never quite get up the energy to do it. Many know their lives could be something more, yet they're sitting in front of the tube, eating junk food, depriving their minds and bodies of the fuel they need to spark new growth."

Furthermore, there are many others who had addressed their weight problems in the past and ended up with failure. They had finally realised how much effort and hard work it takes to lose weight, and just don't have the dedication and determination required to succeed. As a result, they had given up trying to lose weight and had accepted their fate, no matter how deleterious the results. Another reason advanced, though controversial, is that people unconsciously become overweight to protect themselves from others. When you are overweight, you do tend to become 'invisible' and people generally tend to leave you alone. This explanation may be a bit apocryphal, but some people accept this explanation without question. Other reasons for retaining overweight bodies are based on cultural, medical, psychological, environmental and even professional reasons. For example, in movies, some actors and actresses have gained key roles because of their 'bulky' figure.

However, many of you reading this book may not be carrying an enormous amount of weight, but chances are you have some loved ones who have chosen to ignore this problem. It is your duty to provide them with positive reasons as to why they should lose weight before it turns into a matter of life and death. Be careful not to pressurise anyone into undertaking weight reduction measures. It will be more productive if the person under review is given the leeway to make the final decision on whether or not to participate in the Journey.

If you go for a walk into cities and towns in Australia, you will most probably notice thousands of people displaying bodies that carry excess weight, and who are oblivious to prying eyes of the public. So, when you start putting on weight, bit by bit, you might not catch these prying eyes, since you appear similar. This is especially true if your parents, siblings and other relatives are also overweight. You only get noticed once your bulge becomes pronounced.

Why is this indifference to obesity? The short answer appears to be the fear of discussing one's ballooning obesity to others, as others who do not suffer from this problem may make fun of the obese person in front of others. Also, denial is a very powerful tool in dealing (or not) with such problems, and, in any case, it often works very well for a short period of time. It can however be a bridge over short periods of instability that either resolve by themselves or are easier to handle once the initial shock passes away. Additionally, people don't like to think of themselves as having problems, so they feel better about themselves as long as they can ignore them. Denial should be avoided at all costs, but for some sufferers this will be difficult to bypass because the problem may be a difficult one that will open bad emotions. I personally feel that problem-people should be encouraged to solve their own problems at their own pace, and others should concentrate on solving their own problems rather than heaping scorn and ridicule on people facing obesity — because these people need understanding and compassion to overcome their problems. What right do people have to belittle obese people when there is no guarantee the commentators themselves will not become the victims of obesity later in life? I believe that these people should solve their own problems first before belittling and humiliating others.

Contemplation

Corpulent people spend a lot of time thinking about losing weight. They entertain the possibility of undertaking change when they realise that they currently face a problem or might face one in the future. However, a lot of these people are surrounded by uncertainty. They seem to sit in the middle and are not sure whether to commit themselves to a weight loss regime or not. They spend a lot of time looking for information on health and weight loss but are unable to decide if they want to go ahead to bring positive changes to themselves. Generally speaking, people facing weight issues continually attempt to reduce weight, and fantasise about how bright their future will be as a result of the reduction. But, unless they actually go out and seriously do something about it, their dreams will just remain a nonentity.

The Joy of Not Being Fat

"I need to be fat. I am still the same person I was then, but the world is much kinder to me now."
(Unknown).

I came across this quote a while ago and remembered how it perfectly summed up my own personal experience of being a fat person. The truth is, even though I have been overweight for the most part of my life, there have been moments when I have managed to lose a lot of weight temporarily due to sickness. While not being an ideal situation to be in, it has however provided me with the opportunity to live life through the lens of a non-overweight person. It has given me a glimpse of what being lean has to offer and is the major reason why I have spent so many years desperately trying to lose weight.

During these brief moments when my weight was under control, I came to realise how differently people treated me when I was not overweight. Back in the days at the university, I had lost a considerable amount of weight due to the effects of Crohn's disease. It was during this time that I realised how different the world had suddenly turned towards me. Students at my university wanted to hang out with me. I was treated with more respect and received a lot of social invitations. Girls even started flirting with me, which is something I rarely experienced when I was overweight. I remember there was a girl in one of my tutorial classes. I only knew her by face and believed I might have been completely 'invisible' to her. We never spoke to each other. When the semester ended, we all went on Christmas holidays. This is when my Crohn's disease flared up, causing a sudden loss of my weight. When I came back to the university the following semester break, my physical appearance was completely different. I felt like a changed man, as if my past had automatically erased itself from my memory. While sitting at the library, I noticed the same girl who was in my tutorial class in the previous semester, giving me eye contact and later sitting next to me. I was so surprised to find that she suddenly wanted to know me. I do not think she knew I was the same guy in her tutorial class in the previous semester. Subsequently, I felt that my weight loss had changed my overall personality and appearance, boosted my confidence, and enhanced my social skills by leaps and bounds. The conclusion that I reached at that stage was that a good-looking figure would lead to better dating opportunities.

During the worst days of my life I wore very large-size clothes, but during temporary weight reduction periods, due to whatever reason, normal size clothes fitted me comfortably. Prior to getting some peace in life, I always wore baggy clothes to hide fat all over my body. I hated my protuberant stomach. When normal size clothes started to fit my body, I felt so peaceful and relaxed, constantly looked at myself in the mirror and smiled instead of scrutinising myself and letting it affect my mood and tranquility.

When I was young and just started high school, I remember that I could not find school uniforms that fitted my body, and my mother used to take me to the tailor to stitch school uniforms befitting my body. I felt so embarrassed having had to go to the tailor following my mother that later I begged her to take all the relevant measurements at home and then pass the details to the tailor. These days, with the weight problem behind me, I love walking to any drapery shop to buy any clothes that I like. Now I possess a better range of clothes that I could use to enhance my personal appearance and sex appeal.

After I had completed my Journey, I felt so comfortable just wearing a shirt. When I was overweight and my belly was hanging out, I made sure that I wore a T-shirt under my shirt to suppress my belly. I even recall that once in the summer months I wore a jacket to the beach and swam. I felt very embarrassed to be in this "swimming wear" and my friends were yelling at me to take it off. I gave them the excuse that I was feeling cold.

If there was anything I hated more than my big stomach was my large man boobs. Some boys in my school eventually noticed these and started to pinch them. I got teased mercilessly over it. It became such a problem that once I took a bandage and wrapped it around my upper chest section so that my man-boobs would not stick out as much when I went to school. I loved my life so much when I was slimmer and did not have large boobs.

After having completed my weight loss Journey, I became very comfortable in taking walks especially during the day time. Earlier, I hated walking during the day because I did not want people to see me exercising with a huge body, and waited till it was dark. During my walks, I avoided busy roads and chose side streets; I hated busy roads because I did not want drivers to see me walking, and if I ever saw someone walking towards me from the other end of the footpath, I immediately crossed the road to be on the other side to avoid that person.

These are only a glimpse of the mental torture that I experienced during my Journey to fight obesity. But once I successfully overcame this curse of obesity, my lifestyle began to change positively. I felt good about myself and enjoyed my daily life more. My life had changed for the better. I was not worrying or stressing over insignificant things or doing silly things to disguise my flaws. I finally breathed properly and enjoyed myself. My initial health problems forced me to undertake change as I wanted to live my life to the full extent.

Need to Lose Weight

When I was slim I felt as if I was at the top of the world. There is no doubt that life is definitely better when a person is not obese. I had a lot of difficulties struggling with my weight issues and I do not wish to see any person getting into my situation. I was ridiculed, humiliated, suffered from depression, lost direction in life, lost my self-esteem and felt every minute that life was not worth living. Thus, my entire life was preoccupied with my weight. I took all the extreme ways to hide this problem, but at the end of my Journey I am enjoying my life as one should always do.

By addressing my weight issues at an early age and having achieved my goal of reducing my weight, I have gained the following results:

+ Increased self-esteem and confidence;
+ Positive body image;
+ Better social life;
+ More dating opportunities;
+ Better sex life;
+ Less visits to the doctor;
+ No medication required for my Crohn's Disease;
+ No more issues about clothes;
+ No more feeling of shame and worthlessness, and the most important of all,
+ My weight does not control my life any more. I am the master of my own body.

If you are suffering in life due to corpulence and wish to lose weight, then it is time that you make an irreversible decision to fight this disease. Thinking, reading and researching about weight loss will not actually make you lose weight. You will need to take concrete actions and there is no better time to act than now.

What Losing Weight Will Not Do For You

Remember that by losing weight a person will not receive magical powers, nor appear irresistible to men or women, nor solve life's other mundane problems that are not related to obesity. It will not turn one's life into a state of permanent bliss. The variety of sad emotions you experience today may continue to exist even after recovery. So, weight-losing initiatives will address only a small portion of your overall life. You will still have to go to work, put out the garbage bins and participate in a wide gamut of social and economic activities, for example. All or some of these issues may cause you to feel sad, unhappy, irritated, annoyed, etc. But these feelings are not related to your weight, so you cannot expect to lose weight by fighting them.

Another point to remember is that the current state of our health is determined by our composite lifestyle. If you smoke cigarettes or drink excessive amounts of alcohol, losing weight will not help you overcome these issues. You will need to address these issues separately.

Finally, ensure that you do not believe that losing weight will help you find a romantic partner, get a job promotion or get people to treat you with respect. While losing weight can certainly help in these areas, there is no guarantee of success. As for me, I started the weight-loss exercises with low expectations and without attaching specific outcomes; but the final results have been awesome. What I have achieved can also be achieved by another person, but remember that any weight reduction Journey will not end happily. On the other hand, there are millions of overweight people on this earth moving on with their lives with the wrong notion that "things will make me happy." Surely, there are many things that can make life more fun and comfortable for such people in the short run, but a person with a big body will rarely enjoy happiness in the long term. Too often corpulent people seem to focus on the symptoms of obesity instead of examining more deeply the real causes of the issue. If, for example, a person can't fix what is going on inside the body, no external events (e.g. a promotion) or luck (e.g. win in a lottery) will be of much assistance in any weight loss initiative. This is so because the problem may be rooted deeply in culture, psychology, sociology, heredity, etc. In fact, the emotional upheaval caused by weight loss can be devastating. Television, magazines, the internet, and even some health care practitioners lead us to believe that once we lose weight, everything will get better. While it's true that weight loss can boost one's physical and mental state, its emotional consequences, especially for those who have lost considerable weight (e.g. 100kg), are often overlooked. This phase of the weight loss plan should not be ignored and must become part of the overall recovery plan if a person is to remain happy over a longer period.

Is it Too Late for Me to Embark on My Journey?

If you are wondering whether or not it is too late to embark on a weight reduction Journey, then I want to assure you that it is never too late. You should never let your age act as a barrier to success and you should make every effort to improve the quality of your lifestyle for the remainder of your life.

I started my weight loss journey during my mid-twenties. It turned out to be one of the best decisions I have ever made. I could have used my Crohn's disease and past experiences as an excuse not to change my lifestyle. I could have just accepted my fate and continued to exist in a haphazard manner. While this would have been an easy route, it undoubtedly would have led me into an unfulfilled and bland life.

I am so happy that I did not allow my age as a barrier in losing weight. By reducing my weight my philosophy of life has changed tremendously. Now I feel so peaceful and a real human being every day, an outcome that I never expected before enrolling in my weight reduction Journey.

If I knew beforehand that I could achieve my weight loss goals and how happy my life would be in its aftermath, I would have enrolled in the program without question much earlier. Unfortunately, we do not have access to future scenarios so we really do not know what impact change will have on our lives. It is only in the aftermath that one could experience the results – either positive or negative.

If you are in your forties, fifties and even sixties, adopting a healthier lifestyle and addressing your weight problems will ensure that you are living the best life possible for that age. So, never feel that it is too late. Get out there, and start doing something about your weighty problem.

Is It too Late for Me to Lose Weight

If the previous chapter has not convinced you as to why it is never too late to be on your weight loss Journey, let me use a simple arithmetical calculation to convert you. Before I continue, I wish you to bear in mind that to succeed in attaining your weight loss objectives, you have to set aside a few hours every day over a time period ranging from a few months to over three years, depending upon the severity of your problem and the depth of your motivation.

Let us assume that you are currently thirty-five years old and that you will live until the age of seventy. This gives you thirty-five years of life. Suppose at the age of thirty-five you begin your weight loss Journey and that a crude calculation allows you two years to successfully implement your weight programme. If you faithfully dedicate two years of your life to achieving your weight loss goals, then you will be left with thirty-three years to enjoy a healthy and valuable future life. Now, two years may sound like a long time; however, you must realise that it is only 6% of your remaining life. This means that you will still have 94% of your life remaining after only two years of 'apprenticeship' without any worry about weight or being impacted by the other issues that are associated with this condition. I would never consider the age or mindset of a person to be a serious barrier in getting started. My own weight loss Journey began around the age of twenty-nine, and never once did I feel that I was too old or that it was too late for me to get started. By using the above arithmetical calculation, I convinced myself that I still had long years to live and that a few years of sacrifice was worth the investment in time.

You can also try this simple calculation using your own age. Make sure to allocate at least minimum of two years for achieving your weight-loss goals.

Weight Loss Surgery is Not the Answer

An overweight person may opt to undergo a weight loss surgery, such as Lap Band, Laparoscopic Sleeve Gastrectomy, or Laparoscopic Gastric Bypass. While the above options may be suitable for individuals who are morbidly obese and severely suffering from this health issue, or are unable to maintain a healthy body weight despite receiving assistance from medical specialists, for the majority of us, weight-loss surgery is simply not the best option. Surgery is not suitable for people whose diet and lifestyle are out of control. High costs may also preclude many people to opt for surgery. However, the most important reason weight loss surgery is not the answer to fight obesity is because it does not eliminate the root cause of weight gain, and hence may not stop somebody regaining weight after surgery. This is why it is important to first address the root cause of obesity instead of opting for a short cut escape.

Don't Wait for That "Magic Moment" to Get Started

Before embarking on a weight loss Journey, one must wait for the perfect time for the implementation of the plan. This point is very important because a major requirement for people joining a weight reduction program is that their circumstances and surroundings should always be free from distractions of any type. Inevitably, circumstances can change once the initial step is taken, but such negativities should be hidden behind the mind. An example of this is the New Year's resolution. How many times have we heard people say that they will go on a strict diet after the New Year, only to find that their busy lifestyle suddenly creeps upon them after the holiday season, with the result that they will never fully implement their weight loss plan, or even get started.

One of the most popular reasons people give for procrastination is that their busy lifestyle does not allow them to allocate an adequate amount of time to this very important health activity, and that they will actively participate once they find time in the future. Truly, in today's busy society, our free time continually gets taken up by someone or something and no matter how long we continue to wait, that magic moment we seek to begin our nascent weight loss Journey never seems to arrive. Even if we think that we have found that sweet spot in life, further changes in our lives can disrupt your current and future plan. Notwithstanding, once the perfect time to start your weight loss Journey does finally arrive, I can assure you that this magic moment will not last, and that you will find yourself distracted by something else very soon afterwards. I had spent my late twenties just waiting for the right time to start my weight loss Journey. I told myself that I would start once I had completed my studies.

When that was over and as soon as I found a job and started to work from home, then my Journey began seriously. Even then, I periodically found myself in situations that interrupted my weight loss schedule.

You must give obesity and your health the highest priority, and get started as soon as possible. If necessary, you should make changes to your weight loss plan to accommodate your continually changing life circumstances. However, do not delay the start-up process and do at least something to "keep the engine warm and moving."

You Should Ask for Help

If you are having trouble getting started or are unsure when to begin, then you might like to refer to a number of available resources that will help you to prepare, plan and implement your plan. Even though you may feel that you are physically and mentally ready to start the Journey, you may still need additional help. Remember that at the start-up phase you should jettison all your knowledge about losing weight and commit your thoughts to how to lose weight. If you want to reach a certain destination, you will have to take the first steps to get there and others can help you to some extent in your endeavour. You may also like to speak to people close to you for motivation and help in taking the first few crucial steps. Even if they walk with you for a few days, it is likely to boost your confidence and energise you into action. If you have active people in your social circle, assess if you can associate with them and go and participate in a few activities.

One of the best strategies that you may employ at the initial stage is to talk to people around you who had lost weight and ask them how they prepared themselves before starting their Journey.

Find out how long they were thinking about losing weight and what finally made them to actively commit to losing weight. In my case, it was my failing health that set me in motion to take remedial action.

If you have a medical condition or disability that is stopping you from action, make an appointment with your local doctor and see if he/she can provide guidance or perhaps even refer you to a specialist who has shown an interest in treating human corpulence.

Depending on your circumstances, you may need to book an appointment with a psychologist to understand how to overcome mental barriers, if that is what stops you from action. Even seeking the assistance of a life coach can bring some impetus in starting the Journey. Remember that these individuals have helped thousands of people facing the same or similar issues as yours. These people are experts in their own field and can be helpful. One point to remember is that if you are seeking professional help, you should ensure that you utilise somebody who understands you culturally. There is no point in visiting an expert individual who is not familiar with your local cuisine. Remember that diet plays an important role in losing weight and if a person does not understand what food you eat, he will not be a good resource person compared to somebody who has a good understanding of your culinary culture.

I have received a tremendous amount of help from various sources before and after undertaking my Journey. I had people who walked with me, joined me in the gymnasium and even put me on a motor bike which I had to push. My family, to this day, continues to give me health advice. My final advice to you is that you should not be embarrassed in asking for help from anybody who has shown compassion and empathy towards your problem.

Role of Age in Fighting Weight Gain

Your age will play an important role during your Journey. If you have tried to lose weight in the past and failed, remember that with the passage of time you become a different person in many ways. With increasing age, a lot of people mature and become emotionally stronger. So, you must give yourself another chance to achieve success. It is worth a try.

I remember that when I was a teenager I employed all the knowledge I had on weight reduction. But the greatest challenge I faced was controlling my sugar bingeing. The majority of my meals consisted of high levels of sugar. I used to fill my stomach with these junk foods until I was physically ill. I had little control on this habit no matter how hard I tried.

However, as I grew up and matured, I felt a sudden sense of urgency to sculpt my body if I wanted to enjoy a happy life in the future. I decided there and then that I had suffered enough mental torture and that I should change my lifestyle to achieve my dream body. I decided to launch an all-out war on my obesity. It seemed that my current initiatives were failing me and innovative steps were required. But for some unknown reason I stuck with my current plan with added vigour and was surprised to find how easy it was to stick to the same plan. It was like my mind had suddenly developed and strongly urged me not to fall into a relapse. I had to avoid a relapse because I had limited time to achieve my weight goals.

Furthermore, I was not young anymore and I did not have abundant time to start over again with a new plan. When I hit my late twenties, I ceased drinking alcohol and smoking, and intensely became health-conscious. It was as if I was going through a transition. I had more control over my mind and was ready to undertake this Journey with determination and urgency. Now that I am in my early thirties I am able to resist all types of temptations inimical to my body. Suddenly I gained the strength to reject any food that I felt would add weight to my body. Now I have the discipline and willpower to adhere to my weight loss plan without a miss. I am prepared to overcome any hurdles to succeed. I do not understand why I lacked this fighting spirit in my early twenties. I acknowledge that it is very difficult for a person to exercise self-control especially at a young age. At this phase of life, you are still growing up and are faced with many enjoyable activities, so controlling weight will be the last thing that would register in your mind. If you continuously fail to achieve your weight loss goals, don't be too hard on yourself, especially if you are young. Remember that discipline, willpower and other similar attributes are essential for success and it is very likely that you will acquire these qualities and characteristics with the passage of time. You will need time to master the multifarious skills that are needed to achieve your objectives and goals in life. For example, I was suicidal and depressed in my twenties. I did not know how to react to these issues. But by my thirties, I had gained a lot of knowledge, understanding and experience of human diseases and their treatment. This made me stronger mentally and physically. As they say, knowledge is power. My mind has matured a lot since my teenage years. It has become very resilient and adaptable. If you have given up your weight reduction plan for whatever reason, I urge you to retry. This time you just might be mentally and physically better prepared to face the future challenges.

Preparation: Getting Ready to Undertake Change

In the previous chapters, I discussed the factors that finally made me undertake weight change. I also discussed the factors which motivated me to shift my thoughts about weight change to actually do something to reduce weight.

The remainder of this book assumes that you have already made a commitment to reduce your weight and are ready to prepare a plan of action, stage by stage, to achieve your objectives.

You might be under the impression that you can achieve your weight loss goals only through solid dieting and an exercise program. While there are some merits to this line of thought, my experience has taught me that the best way to achieve and maintain your weight loss transformation is by adopting a permanent healthier lifestyle. It is that simple. Remember that it is your current lifestyle that has caused you to emerge the way you have become. It means that bad habits will need to be replaced by good ones. Changes in your lifestyle will be required, and later I will further discuss this aspect. I've had many successes and failures during the years of the implementation of my plan. During this time, I wanted to produce a plan that had to work. I wasn't going to tolerate a plan that might not work. I wanted to guarantee it. I wanted to have rules that would cover my ass should I fall short of expectations.

Exploring the Root Cause of Your Problem

To get started with your preparation, the first thing you must do is sit down and find the root cause of your issues. You need to find the real reason why you are overweight. You can do this by simply asking yourself: "Why am I overweight?"

It has become increasingly common to hear of individuals who are dangerously obese and carrying so much extra weight that they are unable to leave their bed. You have to wonder how on earth they let their weight become such a problem. Yet, the fact that this is no longer an unusual occurrence indicates that there is more at work than simple gluttony. Obviously, eating too much and doing too little physical activities will cause a lot of weight increase, but the question is: why do people allow themselves to put on a lot of weight that impedes their ability to lead meaningful lives. Answering this question honestly is very important because if you do not know what is causing you to gain weight, you will not be able to articulate an appropriate response. You may carry out unlimited exercise and diet all the way to heaven and be rewarded with fantastic results, but unless you remove the variable (s) that are causing the weight gain in the first place, you will never truly beat this issue. Your weight could be a symptom of a bigger problem. You must seek to understand it from all perspectives.

As I mentioned in the earlier chapters, to explore my weight problem correctly, I wrote down all the factors that I felt were contributing to my weight gain. After this, I isolated the major contributors which included sugar. Finally, I chose my addiction to sugar as a causal factor to my abnormal weight. This should not have surprised anyone because I loved food that contained a high level of sugar and I had an addiction to it since my baby days, nurtured by my nanny. So, my Journey started with the total elimination of sugar from my diet, although I admit it was difficult to totally achieve this objective all the time. Apart from avoiding sugary food, I had also completely immersed myself in many physical activities. If your diagnosis shows that sugar is the major factor contributing to your weight increase, then try to immediately eliminate all sugary food from your diet. Concurrently, you should also get involved in diversified physical activities. Remember, one panacea will not apply to all individuals as some other factor, such as heredity, could also be the cause of your obesity. Obviously, the path I had chosen to reduce my weight will not be effective in treating heredity-induced obesity.

Goal Setting

Now that you have found the root cause of your obesity, your next step should be to formulate a goal(s) to address this problem. A SMART goal framework (see Figure 4) can assist you in achieving your goals. A SMART goal is one that is specific, measurable, achievable, relevant and realistic and has a specific time frame. It will ensure that you use a structured approach when creating your weight loss plan and that you can monitor and track your progress. It will allow you to break down your entire program into smaller segments, thus making it more achievable and manageable.

Before the beginning of my Journey, I had created several SMART goals to assist me in obtaining my desired results. One of the goals I created was to meet the fitness criteria for joining the Australian Military Air Force Reserves. In 2016, the fitness requirements for joining the Air Force Reserves (not including exceptions) were:

+ 10 Push-ups, 20 Sit-ups (feet held) and a 6.5 Shuttle run core for males, and
+ 4 Push-ups, 20 Sit-ups (feet held) and a 6.5 Shuttle run score for females.

I have used SMART goals, in conjunction with *gamification* (more information on pages 88–96) elements to lose weight.

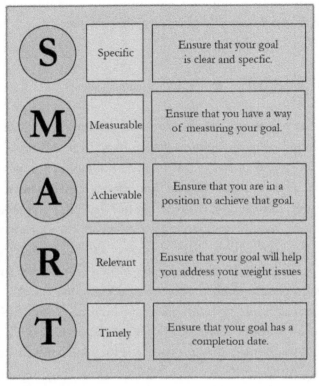

Figure 4 –The S.M.A.R.T goal framework.
(Government of Newfoundland and Labrador 2005)

Here I do not wish to over-emphasise the importance of using a SMART framework to achieve your goals. If you don't use such a tool, chances are you will not be able to monitor the success of your progress in a timely manner.

Dieting

A balanced diet plays a very critical role in fighting obesity. Please do understand that what you are currently putting in your mouth is perhaps the main reason you are in your current situation, unless heredity has been identified as a causal factor. If you are eating too much, you could be eating the wrong types of food. The consumption of the right types of food is likely to reduce your weight. One of the biggest mistakes people make in fighting body weight is to underestimate the importance of a healthy diet and vigorous recourse to physical activities.

Crash diets, quick fixes, and bizarre remedies do not lead to a healthy lifestyle. Slow, steady, and reasonable changes in behaviour do. Theoretically, it is easy to eat less and achieve weight loss. But for many people this is a hugely challenging task especially when they have vague goals and objectives in their plan.

Making Healthier Food Choices and Food Education

"We are digging over our graves with our teeth," wrote the 17th century physician Thomas Moffett (quoted in Robbins, 1997, p.26). Robbins further added: "...we cram our bodies with high fat, nutritionally empty foods, poison our systems with cigarettes, alcohol and drugs, and sit passively in front of our T.V sets."(pp.26-27) These observations suggest that the types of food that go down your throat will have to undergo serious changes. It comes down to this common sense: if the foods you are currently eating is causing your waistline to expand, then you need to change what you are digesting. During my Journey, I was able to swallow a gracious amount of food without gaining weight by making small and smart changes to my diet.

To successfully change your diet, firstly you must list all the food you eat and which food in your opinion is horribly responsible for your weight situation. You need to start treating your

47

body as an engine and your food as a source of fuel. There are many instances of reporting in newspapers of cars either stalling, or jerking or stopping altogether after the filling of petrol. The main reason for these outcomes: adulterated petrol. Similarly, your body needs the right types of fuel (healthy food) to enable all the parts of your body to function efficiently. If you adulterate your body 'fuel' with excessive sugar and fatty food, your body engine is bound to react adversely. With this analogy resting at the back of your mind, you must immediately provide your body with the best fuel (food) possible, food that is high in vitamins and minerals. Consumption of high quality foods will ensure that our body is not starving for nutrition.

Thus, food education should become an integral component of your weight loss plan. In this regard, you will have to develop an interest in understanding where your food comes from and how your body responds to it. Based on the information that you have obtained, you should make necessary changes to your eating behavior, which should exclude sugary and fatty food. However, if you continue to gain weight despite avoidance of these types of foods, then look for healthier alternatives. If required, read the food labels and the ingredients on the food label. During my Journey, if I could not pronounce an ingredient on the food label of a product, I did not consume it. Obviously, this was an overreaction, but at times people in a desperate situation usually make silly decisions.

Learning more about the foods you enjoy eating is a good starting point before making adjustments to your diet. Before I commenced my Journey, I wrote down the benefits and disbenefits of each food that was in my pantry. If I discovered a food item that I thought was bad for my waist, I sought a healthier replacement or eliminated it from my diet altogether. One of the first steps I took was to replace all the soft drinks, sodas, and hot beverages with green and Rooibos tea without sugar.

This ensured that I was not putting all artificial ingredients and sugars into my body. It made my life a lot easier. These days, I drink a gracious amount of green tea on a daily basis. Initially all types of tea tasted insipid, but with the passage of time my taste buds adjusted to the taste.

I was also fortunate that my family had a garden that was actively maintained by my father. I added all green leafy vegetables he grew to my diet. It was all natural and organic and tasted good. Fresh vegetables from the supermarkets and other sources do not always taste as good. My father also grew a lot of carrots as well, and I had by far the largest share of it. Converting carrots into juice and drinking it immediately gave me a lot of satisfaction. From that day onwards, I ensured that I had a glass of carrot juice every day. This is perhaps the first time I realised the importance of growing food in the garden. If you are in a position to grow your own food, do not hesitate and get the spade out. Gardening can be a great and productive hobby and consumption of home grown food can assist you greatly in achieving your weight loss goals.

Another change that I made to my diet was to digest a lot of steamy food such as steamed potatoes, sweet potatoes, cassava, green leafy vegetables, carrots and eggs. I realised very early that not only is it relatively easy to steam-cook food but that a person can take a lot more of it without putting on weight.

There is no doubt that dietary changes entail a great deal of personal sacrifices. But any pain caused by the implementation of these changes will be offset by their positive outcomes. Furthermore, once you get used to steam-cooked food you will stick to it, even after you have conquered your obesity.

The Sugar Epidemic

In the earlier chapters, I discussed in detail about my addiction to sugar and my discovery that sugar was the root cause of my obesity. If there is one item I would highly recommend you remove completely from your diet, it is sugar. Based on own personal experience and from my intensive research, I have concluded that sugar is the major cause of the obesity crisis facing the world today. It is the key component that leads to weight gain. Research also has indicated that sugar is a highly addictive substance. It has been compared to cocaine and heroin.

Unfortunately, many of the food we eat on a regular basis contain a lot of sugar. These include items such as:

- White bread
- Bread Spreads
- Chocolates and Biscuits
- Soft Beverages (coffee, chocolate shakes)
- Fast Food
- Soft Drinks
- Food Sauces
- Breakfast Cereals
- Nutrition Bars
- Salad Dressings
- Doughnuts, Muffins and Cakes
- Canned Fruit
- Ice Cream
- Potato Chips
- Table Sauces

All these food items will certainly contribute to weight gain, especially if a person has a habit of binge eating. Unfortunately, I had fallen into the trap to binge eat all the above foods at an early age, and the ones with high sugar content were my favourites. As emphasised before, the first step that one must take with utmost urgency is either to avoid eating sugary products altogether or eat sugary food that contain less sugar. It is unfortunate that many people who have had the taste of sugar very early in life would find it difficult live a life without sugar. However, you must get into your consciousness that it is certainly possible to live without a high dosage of sugar.

Whatever conclusions others might reach on the value, or otherwise, of sugar consumption, my personal experiences have convinced me that the removal of sugar from my diet has invariably led to the de-escalation of my weight. Not surprisingly, there were some moments in my life when I did not consume high levels of sugar and still lost weight, even without trying.

Giving up sugar and sugary food may sound like a tough challenge, and it certainly is. However, by self-educating yourself on the interaction between sugar and our mind and body, and by creating a strategy to gradually wean away from it, you will ensure a better chance of fighting the sugar epidemic. Any attempt to withdraw from sugar should be seen as withdrawal from drug addiction. Sugar is very addictive and has been designed to create dependency. It must be designated a drug, and we must treat it as a drug. Believe me, once you free yourself from this substance, which is your jail, you will not miss it. If you wean away from sugar, you will always say to yourself: "It was worth it."

Drinking Blended Fruits and Vegetables

One of the most inspirational moments during my Journey was when I watched the movie/documentary "Fat, Sick, and Nearly Dead". This movie provided cogent reasons why people should eat an excessive amount of fruits and vegetables to fight obesity. The ideas presented in this film have since embedded in my mind and I have implemented a large number of them in order to minimise my dependence on food high in sugar. Throwing fruits and vegetables in a blender is one of the easiest ways to get all the vitamins and minerals that our body needs. By actively deriving nourishment from food and vegetables, I do not at all get the feeling that I am starving for nutrition, and now my craving for sugar has diminished. Having a blended fruit juice for breakfast gives me the natural source of sugar I need and ensures that I do not seek out processed sugar options during the day.

Since watching "Fat, Sick, and Nearly Dead", I have developed a passion for drinking different combinations of blended fruits and vegetables. My innovative menus make my body feel healthy and tranquil all the time — day and night. Let me give you a few of my innovative and favourite combinations that I blend regularly. These include:

+ Watermelon, Strawberries and Blueberries
+ Watermelon, Grapes, broccoli
+ Banana, Blueberries, dates
+ Carrots, Soy Milk, Cucumber, Water melon
+ Rock melon, Spinach, Kale, Broccoli.

If you wish to taste my blended juices, beware that one or two menus are very insipid, especially those having a preponderance of vegetables. However, by adding one sweet fruit to the mix (such as watermelon, or banana or oranges) will ensure that the juice becomes more palatable.

One question people frequently ask me is: "Is sugar from fruits bad for your health?" The answer is No. When our bodies absorb natural sugar from fruits, we also consume fibre that come along with them. This ingredient helps counter all the negative effects created by sugar alone. Sugars found in fruits only become a problem when the fibre is removed. Blending ensures that fibre is retained along with all the sugar found in the fruits, so do not be scared to blend fruits.

Nowadays, the blending of fruits and vegetables has become an important activity in my life. After my workout, I blend spinach and kale with fruits and create a post-workout drink. The green leafy vegetables provide me with sufficient protein. If I crave for sugar, I drink a glass of fresh fruit juice instead of grabbing a packet of biscuit. I highly encourage you to give blending a shot by slotting this drink somewhere in your weight loss plan. I have no doubt you will find the result amazing.

Counting Calories

During my weight loss Journey, I browsed through several articles that I discovered online on obesity. The most common theme that I came across in these articles related to the counting of calories. The basic concept of calorie count entails the keeping of a journal on which a person notes the daily consumption of calories, and the need to watch that the daily target is not exceeded. While some people may find this activity interesting in trying to overcome obesity, I, however, never counted calories during my weight loss Journey. I felt it to be inconvenient, a hassle, time consuming, and it did not seem natural to me. Leave aside the flippancy, I never saw my grandparents counting calories, and I doubt our ancestors did the same back in the day in their caves. Calorie-counting seems to be a modern phenomenon. In any case, I was not ready to implement this activity in my plan. By adopting a healthier diet and exercising regularly, I did not feel that there was any need to count calories. My diet consisted primarily of fruits, vegetables, potatoes, rice, fish, meat and fresh produce, and these items, when taken in moderation, are not likely to make people very fat. My food was always prepared in a healthy way and I ate it graciously and without fear of adding on weight. As I mentioned before, the removal of sugar from my diet was the key step in my weight loss strategy, and, as I had originally suspected, excessive consumption of sugar was the main cause of my obese condition.

However, I can understand why professional bodybuilders, athletes and many individuals, who make a living by providing an array of health services, compulsorily count calories particularly in their weight reduction exercises, because participants in these programmes wish to keep a precise account of the calorie loss/gain on a daily basis. Exercisers generally wish to keep a precise record of calories before and after an exercise. Using information gained on calories and weight they are in a better position to assess the effectiveness of their weight loss training. However, for individuals like you and me whose main objective generally is to lose weight and build some muscles, focusing too much on calories could become a major digression.

In any case, it is important to note that the counting of calories is not recommended if you are eating healthy food and follow a disciplined diet. However, if you do want to count calories, first try to remove sugar from your diet and then eat healthy meals and exercise regularly. If you do not see positive results flowing and your weight continues to rise, then there may be a need for further exploration of the root cause of your problem, which could be rooted on some other factor. If you find that the root cause can be resolved by counting calories, then apply this principle to your weight loss strategy. However, do not count calories just for the sake of counting calories or because you have read about it on the internet. Do not clutter your mind with unnecessary activities.

Clearing Your Pantry

Your diet will play an important role in your weight loss Journey, and it is very important that you should get rid of all the unnecessary food from your pantry. These may include biscuits, chocolates, soft drinks and the other junk food. Throw them out! Remember, you are aiming for a total change in lifestyle and your pantry must match the healthier lifestyle that you are aiming to achieve. If you "defiantly" keep these junk food, then it is most likely that instead of making progress you will fall into a relapse whenever you over-attack these junks with your mouth. Your willpower may not be strong enough to resist the temptation to devour this junk food. This means that you should never trust your willpower as a potent weapon against gluttonous impulse. Furthermore, remember that a small amount of willpower is available to us every day and we should not waste it. After a day's hard work or during times of crisis, it is easy to forget your goals and to quickly turn to junk food. Thus, by not having easy accessibility to these types of food in the first place you are taking proactive measures to prevent a relapse.

During my Journey, I used my strong willpower and cleaned out all the junk food out of my pantry. I threw out all the biscuits, soft drinks, hot beverages, sauces, bread spreads and even sugar. Instead, I replaced all these food with nutritional delights such as fruits and vegetables and wholemeal items. Sure, this action may seem extreme and a little boring, but the results had been worth it.

I cannot over-emphasise the importance of a healthy diet. If you can give your body quality nutrition, you do not need to eat junk food. Plus, why would you want to make life hard for yourself by keeping junk food in your house? By getting rid of them and switching to healthier alternatives, you will be in a better position to achieve your weight reduction goals.

Getting Comfortable Throwing Food Away

One of the first lessons I learnt from my parents was that we should not throw away food. I was constantly reminded how there were people in the world who did not have food to eat and how lucky I was that I had plenty food on my plate. It was drilled into me that food was a precious resource and something that we should not waste. It was this type of thinking that led me to eat everything that was presented to me. No matter how full I was, I would always ensure that my plate was empty — even if force was required. I could not bring myself into throwing away food due to regular brainwashing. Of course, this way of thinking not only contributed to my weight gain but also led to a bigger appetite. This gluttony eventually led me into a quagmire from which I eventually had to extricate myself at a great cost.

If you also have similar feelings on throwing away food just as I had, then you immediately need to break that mode of thinking. You must understand that you must eat the amount your body needs, and not what moralists dictate. Sure enough, there are people in this world starving but do not let guilt control you. Understand that it is OK to throw food away if you wish to, but on the other hand, superfluous eating is an example of self-inflicted cruelty indirectly championed by moralists. If you seriously take the advice of these people and overeat instead of throwing away leftover food, it is unlikely these people will treat you with compassion once you become obese. Based on my experience, once you are obese and look 'ugly', you are on your own. Everybody will heap the blame on you for being in the condition you are.

Minimise Overeating

One major mistake I had made early in life was to continually eat until I was stuffed. Unfortunately, my body, though big, did not need all the food that I was digesting. Considering that the types of food that I mostly consumed were usually high in sugar, I found it very difficult to resist the temptation to empty the plate. This unusual eating behaviour ensured that any existing initiative that I had on weight reduction was doomed to failure. Fortunately, I realised at this stage that unless I changed my eating habits, I was never going to succeed in achieving an ideal body weight.

In this context, the important point to remember here is that it takes our body around 15-20 minutes to send a signal to the brain that it is full. Your body knows how much food it needs and you must give it time to do its job. When we do not get that feeling of satiety, we assume that we should eat more. Of course, this is completely wrong. Your body will let you know if you need to eat more or not. This entire process can be a challenging task but you must have faith and trust in it to succeed.

By adopting a good diet that contains a lot of vitamins and minerals you should accelerate loss of your body weight. When you eat healthy foods, your body will not starve for nutrition. If you do not provide the body with the nutrition it needs, you will constantly feel hungry as the body will continue to send you "hungry" signals. That is why a balanced diet is a very important part of our life.

Finally, during my Journey I managed to overcome my gluttonous proclivity with a decent breakfast. A decent breakfast ensured that I did not over-eat later in the day. As I had provided my body with satiety early in the morning, I was able to go longer during the day without food. If I missed lunch or did not have food until I got home, I ensured that I would feed on a vegetable-based meal that was prepared in my kitchen. On some occasions when I skipped breakfast, I would later crave for sugary food and at the earliest opportunity in the afternoon would search for a local supermarket and fill my shopping bag with junk food. However, by having food on a piecemeal basis throughout the day I ensured that I avoided gluttony at the next regular meal. This principle is very important and must be followed. While overeating is bad for health, so is under-eating, which can create many other health problems, such as anorexia which particularly affects younger females. In fighting obesity, I was not scared to eat, but at no time did I over-eat the wrong foods.

These days, I take plenty of fruits and vegetables in all my meals. My eating binge, if it takes place at all, is restricted to these two types of foods. So, I am not worried about overeating fruits and vegetables; the only thing I am worried about is to make a pig of myself.

Starving Yourself

One of the myths perpetuated by many people is that obesity could be fought by 'starving' your body of food. Their rationale is that if you starve your body of the fatty and sugary food, then you are probably on the right path. However, starving your body with all types of food as part of a weight reduction programme will be counterproductive as our survival depends on food consumption. As stated in the previous section, girls particularly wishing to maintain their body image will avoid as much food as they can in the hope of looking skinny and younger. However, those who take such experiments to the extreme are bound to suffer a number of medical problems later in life. The problem of adopting "starvation" as a tool to reduce weight is that a little food now will have to be compensated with a little more food at a later round. If this realisation does not set in early in your mind, then later you will be stuck in a vicious cycle from which an escape would be difficult. In any case, the so-called techniques used in reducing weight, such as "starvation" or "temporary hunger", should never be a part of a sustainable weight reduction plan.

I am sorry to state that at the original stage of my Journey I had employed 'hunger tactic' as part of my plan to reduce weight. In this regard, I took one meal a day expecting to witness a miracle in a few weeks. Surprisingly, miracles did happen, for I noted that I was losing approximately a kilogram of weight every two days. My joy knew no bounds. I felt as if I was at the top of the world. At that time, I was attending university and I could not be fixated on a rigid plan. While adoption of such untested and haphazard plans made sense to me at the educational level, it did not work at the personal level, for any person wishing to seriously confront personal obesity must adhere to a credible weight reduction plan over a longer period.

Because I relied too much on my unreliable 'crazy quilt" methods my progress suddenly came to a halt, for the more I deliberately starved myself the more I had to eat to support my big body. Admittedly, I felt this routine to be psychological torture at its worst. Imagine you feel hungry but because you want to lose weight, you decide not to eat. Is this a good way to lead a happy life? My life was getting messier. I felt that I could not live any longer in this manner. My body started to signal my mind, "please can I have some more." I felt as if I was on the horns of dilemma. I was getting frightened that I was going to die. Luckily, within two weeks' of being on my own plan, I fell into a relapse. In this state, I had no control over any food that was around my house. I cursed my weight reduction plan and I cursed any person who appeared in my mind. My visits to the supermarkets became more often. I carried this behaviour for a few weeks in response to undoing all the past weeks' achievements that were obtained by sheer willpower and perseverance. Later, I regained my health and body back in good condition after adopting a recognised weight reduction plan.

Finally, please take this advice from me: Don't starve yourself to reduce your weight. Eat as much as you like, but eat the right food.

Creating Custom Diets

As I have argued before, a balanced diet is an important component of a weight reduction plan. The diet that I strictly used during my Journey was a custom diet that I concocted by using various ingredients. Similarly, as part of your weight loss goals, you will inevitably have to adopt an anti-obesity diet. There are amazing diet programmes available online that you can adapt or adopt to achieve success during your Journey. These diets have strong community support behind them. Diets such as Atkins, Paleo, Vegan and Fruitarian are popular amongst people facing weight issues, and you may find that at least one or a few of them will meet your needs. You do not need to obsess about going Paleo versus low-fat versus low carb or whatever. Just eat more good food, and less bad food; more veggies and whole, unprocessed foods and less of anything that comes in a box with a logo on it.

However, remember that everyone is different and what works for one person may not work for another. At one time, there was a popular banana diet that appeared on the internet. The basic idea of this diet was simply to eat as many bananas as your body can accommodate. Now, as ridiculous as this diet may sound, it actually worked for some people. There may be some veracity in this story, because a few years ago there was a story in a local TV about a Queensland man who was eating eighty bananas a day. Unbelievably, in the TV picture he looked very lean. On the contrary, there are many skeptics who have found that an excessive consumption of bananas will add more weight to the body. Of course, this does not mean that a banana diet is problematic; it could only mean that it works for some people while not for others. For this reason, it is better to concoct a flexible diet, one that is not only receptive to your body but which meets your personal and cultural requirements. Also, remember that some diets may require you to cook; but do you have the time and resources to cook? Some diets may promote certain food, but are there any cultural barriers that may prevent you from eating it? Some diets are very restrictive, but would it suit your lifestyle?

Remember that diets available online are generic and do not take into account a person's personal situation. That is why it is important for you to ensure that you adopt a diet that meets your particular needs. During my Journey I took bits and pieces of various diets discovered online and then concocted my own custom super diet. This really worked for me as I was able to customise it to suit my particular needs. I suggest you should also make an effort to experiment with various diets and create one that helps you in fighting your weight problem. Obviously, you will need several trial and error experiments before discovering an ideal diet.

You Should Not Entertain "Cheat Days"

It is common to read about individuals who have added "cheat days" to their weight loss strategy. Cheat Days are days when a person can eat anything, and these usually include food that they had previously been prevented from eating. While many people support the idea of cheat days, I am against it as I have found it to be one of the quickest ways to fall into a relapse. A cheat day may look promising on paper, but it is a trap. As I have discovered during my own Journey, having a cheat day can be very destructive. When I embarked on my Journey, I decided to have a weekly cheat day to satisfy my sugar cravings. However, what I eventually realised was that while the mood was good during the actual day, the subsequent days were filled with guilt, anger and misery. I felt as if I had taken a huge leap backwards. The fact that I could eat anything I wanted also ensured that my body took a massive hit, thus requiring a few days to recover. This severely affected my ability to continue with my weight loss routine. Another problem that I faced was that on the day following the cheat day, I would concoct various excuses and tactics to participate in another cheat day — another day to indulge, binge and elevate my mood. Luckily, I did not succumb to these temptations quite often; if I had, I would have definitely fallen into a relapse and later embroiled into the quagmire of a vicious cycle – triggering of my brain to revert to my previous mischievous eating habits and my fresh attempts to gain traction - a very dreadful scenario for any person.

The avoidance of falling into a relapse after a cheat day was a very traumatic moment in my life. However, I am not certain if I had enough stamina in reserve to avoid repetition of this phenomena over a longer period of time. In any case, subsequently, I removed cheat days from my weight reduction strategy. I could not afford nor risk going into a relapse and undoing all the hard work and effort that I had already put into my anti-obesity plan.

Despite what has been my experience about cheat days, Dr Oz of the TV fame has another viewpoint. According to him:

Tons of dieting experts agree that you should build in "cheatdays" since too much deprivation can actually lead to more cravings, causing you to break from your diet. In addition, going off your diet once in a while stimulates the thyroid gland and can "wake up" your metabolism. Cheating in a sensible way will help steer you toward success in the long-term. (http://www.doctoroz. com/print/44349).

As an alternative to the cheat days, I indulged in a high quality, nutrition-filled meals consisting mostly of fruits and vegetables. I found this to be an ideal substitution as it allowed me to eat larger quantities of meals, whenever I wanted, without facing any negative consequences. By avoiding unhealthy foods on a long-term basis, I also ensured that my body was able to adapt to a healthier diet.

While you are on your Journey, I want you to think carefully whether or not you wish to exploit cheat days. It is understandable that some of you cannot avoid your favourite dishes and thus may readily opt for cheat days. Watch out, it will be heart breaking to fall into a relapse and watch months of progress go into waste. Remember that you gave up unhealthy food for a reason, which was to lose weight. Please do not let go off this idea.

Finally, I have now learned to live without the junk food that I used to eat, and I believe you can do the same. Our body takes a while to adjust to different food intakes and I am convinced your body will respond kindly to any change in your food intake. I also do not miss eating junk food anymore as I feel that I have already eaten my life's quota. However, I have promised myself that my food indulgence would restart when I am seventy years old. Until then, it is all about eating 'clean' food and achieving my post weight- loss goals.

Beginning to Exercise

Do you hate exercising? Well, start loving it. Exercising will play an important role in your weight-loss Journey as it facilitates the creation and implementation of an exercise routine in your weight loss plan to accelerate the fat burning process. I understand that a lot of people hate exercising. It appears to be a necessary evil, but it has to be done.

If you are unsure where to begin regarding exercising, you can get the ball rolling by simply going for a walk. This is how I got started. I found walking to be a very easy, affordable and a convenient activity, and lost a lot of weight by walking regularly. It was ideal for a beginner. As I got more serious about my health and my goals became clearer, I added weight lifting to my routine.

You can find a lot of beginner's information on walking on the internet, especially information related to medical prerequisites, footwear technique, and finding good walking tracks designed by your local council. If you possess a similar personality to mine and find walking the same routes boring, you can always add a bit of variety by creating different walking routes. There is no need to take the same route every day. Find a map of your local area and start exploring all the walking paths. You could use this opportunity to find a bit more about your neighbourhood. For example, if your search shows that there is a park near your house, then perhaps you might want to add jogging to complement your walking routine.

I love walking. It is my favourite hobby. However, there is one thing I hate about walking and it is the return walk. A return walk is a route where you simply walk from point A to point B, and return the same way. It usually becomes boring as you are walking the same route twice in one session, so I always try to find a route that allows me to walk in a circle. I have a policy that apart from my home street, I will never walk on the street twice during a session. I always try to walk in a circle. If you decide to add walking to your exercise routine and make significant progress in your battle to lose weight, you could further challenge yourself by walking with body weights. This is how I went about adding intensity to my walks, to make it more challenging. At one stage, I was walking with a bag full of books and later threw in some weight plates. If this does not work for you, there are also professionally-made body weight options available on the market.

However, by the time I finished walking with weights, my legs were 'dead'; it was a thorough workout.

One of the drawbacks of walking was that your plan could be affected by rain, cold weather and a lot of other factors. There were numerous occasions during my Journey when I could not go for a walk because of bad weather which killed my momentum. Because bad weather is beyond my control, I did manage to address this issue by purchasing a home gym.

Despite these minor drawbacks, I feel that walking is still a great way to start the fat burning process. If you make a commitment to walk 45 minutes to an hour daily, 5 times a week, you will be well on your way to successfully completing your lifestyle change.

Remember this: If you try to reduce your weight only by exercising, then it is important that you keep in mind the distinction between health and fitness, as both do not mean the same. Robbins (1991: 440-41) makes the distinction between these two words as follows:

Fitness is the "physical ability to perform athletic activity."
Health is...defined as "the state where all the systems of the body—nervous, muscular, skeletal, circulatory, digestive, lymphatic, hormonal, etc.-are working in an optimal way...."
So, when you go to a gym with a view to trimming your weight,

you will in fact be more dedicated to fitness and less to health. Health suggests maintaining a harmonious functioning of all the major organs of the human body, and the benefits of this are not immediate but will flow evenly as you age. As a matter of fact, both types of activities are beneficial, but if you give more preference to fitness over health, then you may not live long to enjoy your well-sculpted body (Robbins, 1992).

Street-Walking and Feeling Self-Conscious

If you are obese, have you ever found yourself in a situation where you were walking on the street during your exercise and then noticed another person approaching you from the other side and you cross the road to avoid that person?

While walking has generated solid results for me, the biggest problem I initially faced was to remain self-conscious while walking on the streets. I felt wrongly that people on the street were staring and laughing at me, at my bulky figure, and were against my exercising in general. It is very difficult to explain such a painful feeling to somebody who has not experienced it, but those who have will empathise with me. As the result of this experience, I usually waited until the evening to go walking so that I could use the nighttime to exercise in secrecy. But fear of robbery and violence curtailed my nocturnal exercising to a great extent, exacerbated further by attending a number of social obligations and bad weather. Nowadays I walk anytime during the day without feeling self-conscious. It did take a bit of effort to change my thinking, but I managed to get there.

Below are some tips to help you maintain your momentum should you face the issues that I had encountered:

+ The people you see while out walking during the day

are too occupied with their own life to worry about you or how you look;

+ If people who are exercising notice you, remember that they might be worried about their own flaws and more concerned about you judging them;

+ When you are walking on a busy road and there are plenty of cars on the road, consider that people who see you might actually be happy that you are making an effort to do something about your health and might even be inspired;

+ I found that walking with a school bag helped. This was to give people the impression that I was going to school or work instead of exercising. As result, I was less worried about people seeing me exercise. This was a pure psychological fraud that worked very well for me.

+ I also found wearing large sized clothes helpful as it covered up the areas I was self-conscious about; and finally

+ I kept a positive attitude and continued to tell myself that tomorrow would not be as hard as today, and that the more weight I lost, the easier walking would become, and that one day I would not have to worry about this issue.

While the above tips can provide you with some sort of relief, only by losing weight will you be able to overcome the issue of self- consciousness.

Once my weight went down, I automatically felt over-confident walking on the street. In fact, I found it amusing when I noticed other people crossing the streets walking towards me when they saw me walking towards them.

However, you will have to overcome and put aside whatever irrational thoughts that initially arise, and just go out and walk. It will get easier once your body fat starts burning.

Starting to Lift Weight

Adding a weight lifting regime to your workout is an excellent way to burn extra calories and start building muscle. Having a strong and muscular physique will add to your confidence. The last thing you would want to become is "skinny fat". I have a weight lifting regime in place as part of my strategy. It is nothing fancy, but delivers the results that I wished to achieve.

I mentioned earlier that I have a home gym. These are the equipment that I have in my gym:

+ A Treadmill
+ Bench Press
+ Olympic barbell
+ Weight plates (2 x 20, 2 x 10, 2 x 5, 2 x 2.5, 2 x 1.25)
+ Stretching Mat.

The biggest challenge that I initially faced was not so much as acquiring these items but finding a place to locate them. The last thing I wanted was to invest in a gym that I could not use. But when my dad saw my tremendous enthusiasm in weight-loss initiatives he made available to me a large room which I quickly converted into a gym. If you are unsure about investment in a home gym, you should first go to your local gym until such time you have a gym of your own. In any case, you will only need a gym if you have a passion for weight lifting. In my case, my love for my home gym is so deep that I cannot imagine ever joining a public gym. If you decide to add a lifting routine to your exercise, ensure you seek medical advice first and educate yourself about nutrition and how to lift the weight correctly. This will ensure that you maximise muscle gain and prevent injuries.

One important point to remember when you use a home gym is that you should have long-term or strategic goals in mind when you begin to lift weight. You should also be very clear about answers to questions such as what do you want to achieve within the timeframe you have set. You should never start working on a gym hardware without proper direction. Many people who have drastically reduced their weight using gym exercises have found employment as:

+ Bodybuilder
+ Powerlifter
+ Sports Athlete
+ Military Personnel

Each of the above type of people, though possessing overlapping skills, has a different approach and produces different outcomes in providing their services. They perform much better because they follow prescribed goals and objectives and strictly adhere to the correct workout plan to assist their clients.

I chose power lifting to build my body strength and size. To achieve these goals without facing much hurdles, I created a custom workout plan based on the 5x5 strong lifts workout program. As my goals and ambitions were different from others at that time, I did my own research and came up with my customised workout plan. It was very unlikely that my setup would have suited the needs of many others, just as a workout plan designed by others would not have met my needs. Thus, you should carry out your own research and choose the best workout plan that suits your needs, rather than basing your exercising on the plan devised by another person. If you are a gym enthusiast, I highly recommend that you keep on adding weights to your weight lifting exercise routine. In this way, you will be able to assess periodically whether you are gaining power in your body or not.

Sacrificing Your Time for Exercise

After exercising for an hour in the morning, I felt wonderful and got energised by adopting a positive mindset. I do understand many of you, for various reasons, would not be able to sacrifice an hour daily on exercising. However, let's examine this setup so you can see it from a different perspective.

There are 24 hours in a day. I sacrifice one hour daily on exercises. I feel blissful in the remaining 23 hours.

Let me now convert these into percentages:

- 1 hour a day = approximately 4% of my day exercising.
- 23 hours in a day = 96% feeling awesome.

So here I have the option of sacrificing around 4% of my day to feel happy around 96% of the time. I believe this is a great trade off and, depending on your goals, you may not even need to sacrifice an hour a day but even less, to feel great. The important thing to realise here is that you will have to make enormous sacrifices to achieve your goals. These may entail a great sacrifice of your time, perhaps the foods you love to eat and even the activities you enjoy in order to make progress towards your weight loss goals.

Having a Rest Day

Rest days are very important for a healthy living, so do not underestimate the need for taking a break from your exercise routine. Remember that you build muscles when you are resting. You must give your body the opportunity to undergo the repairing process.

One of the early mistakes I made during my weight-loss Journey was to exercise every day. At times, I would exercise for 14 to 17 days in a row. Now I realise that this was certainly an over-kill.

When you first start to exercise, your weight tends to come down a lot quicker. I used to lose around half a kilo every day. As a result, I used to love exercising daily just to see the weight come down fast. However, eventually the weight would stop coming down fast. This is the point where the newbie weight loss ends and it suddenly takes longer to lose weight. I felt that I was not training hard enough and pushed myself harder, only to exhaust myself and eventually falling into a relapse.

Another reason I hated to take rest days was because of the feeling that I would over-eat during the day and then end up putting back a lot of weight. This feeling is very similar to the scenario when you blow out your diet and then feel like throwing in the towel. If I went two to three days without exercise, I suddenly felt overweight and as if I had undone many months of training. Obviously, such feelings are psychological in nature, but, nevertheless, a constant source of worry. However, this changed a few years later when I decided that I would juggle my exercise routine due to time constraints. I decided that I would exercise every alternate day — one day exercising and the other day resting. Even though I felt that I was not doing enough, I managed to stick to this routine for a month. Towards the end of the month, I had a family gathering. To my surprise, all my relatives commented on my lean figure. I was shocked. This was because I had thought all along that I was not going to lose much weight because I took many rest days and the results were the opposite. It was at this stage when I got convinced that there was no need for me to exercise every day.

These days, I ensure that I rest at least 3 days a week. I give the body a break from all the lifting. If I do feel the itch to exercise, I usually go for a light walk. However, I do ensure that I have days where I do some form of exercise. In any case, if you still wish to exercise regularly do remember that you will not make much progress unless you give your body a bit of timeout. Your body needs time to rest, repair and recover. If you push yourself too hard, you will become exhausted and may throw in the towel. It is vital you take some resting days to ensure that you still have the strength and vitality to maintain an exercise routine for a longer period. So, no matter how bad you feel during your rest days, please do realise that you are one step closer to achieving your desired weight goals.

Role Models For Inspiration

When I initially started lifting weights, I frequently looked up to celebrities, fitness gurus and social media health personalities for guidance and inspiration. As these individuals were accomplished in their fields, I felt that they would have a tremendous amount of experience to share, and that their knowledge and experience would help me attain my goals. So, I subscribed to their channels and newsletters, and religiously listened to the advice that they offered. However, it did not take me long to lose my interest in these people. You see, while they were motivational, the advice that they were giving was not addressing the lifestyle that I was aiming for. I did not have any aspirations of having a body like a bodybuilder. I was not interested in that "beast" look. All I wanted was to become a lean, fit and muscular-looking individual — nothing over the top.

You will find that individuals who seriously look up to celebrity bodybuilders are professionals who work within the industry, or want to compete in competitions. These guys usually operate on a different level. They train for a living. It is a bread and butter job for them. They were not very useful to me, however. I was just an ordinary guy who just wanted to lose weight, get my diet in shape and build some muscles.

Nevertheless, I learnt one important lesson from these celebrities, and that was to associate with those role models who had similar lifestyles and goals as I possessed. So, I isolated individuals who were vegan bodybuilders, cyclists and individuals who provided nutritional and spiritual advice. They were completely different from the professional bodybuilders.

The important lesson that I learnt was that when you start listening to advice given by your fellow men, make sure that the person in question promotes the lifestyle you are aiming for. There is no point following the advice and workout programs that professional bodybuilders recommend when you only want to lose weight and shape your body. Remember that these people are brands and they make money by selling their services. Worse still, they may not even use the items they promote and recommend workouts that require supplements. All their activities revolve around cleverly marketing their products and services and maximising their profits.

So, when you pick a role model, please ensure that you find somebody who meets your particular needs. In my case, the role models who brought changes to my life were teachers of spirituality and alternative health.

Membership in a Gymnasium

When it comes to losing weight and building muscles, one of the first considerations that normally should come into a person's mind is whether or not to join a gymnasium (gym). There is no doubt that by following a solid gym routine, a person can achieve wonderful body transformation, especially when a diverse range of equipment and services can be accessed at the same time.

However, the question that I wish to pose is — do you REALLY need a gym membership? The reason I have brought this question up is because I have had great success with a small home gym, and you may prefer to take this route. The benefits of having a gym at home are huge and I prefer working out here instead of at my local gym whose membership fees may be outside the ambit of many working people. Let me give you my reasons why I advocate a home gym:

+ Cost: I was able to purchase my entire home gym for approximately $1200 Australian dollars. This was a one-off investment, which paid itself off within 14 months. I am now saving money.

+ Solitude. I am one of those people who enjoys exercising in solitude. When alone, I have less distractions and I can fully concentrate on my weightlifting and achieve better results. My local gym is usually full of distractions and this seriously affects my momentum and ability to complete a solid workout. These distractions are non-existent when I exercise in isolation at my home gym.

+ Clothing: At my home gym, I can wear any type of cloth during workouts. Sometimes, I might also put on a gym outfit which I might wear 3 - 4 times before washing. At home, I really do not have to worry about wearing unwashed clothes. This just makes life easier. When it comes to the local gym, you need to be considerate about not offending others with smelly clothes, and I personally do not have the time to wash and wear fresh clothes to the gym to please others.

+ Convenience: My gym is just a yard away from my bedroom. When your gym is that close, there are less obstacles and barriers in getting there. When it comes to going to my local gym, I need to wear proper clothing, pack a bag, drive to the gym, check-in, wait for the machines to be free, and adhere to gym rules, all of which can give you many reasons to give it a miss. With my home gym though, it's just about walking next door, putting on clothes and getting on with the programme. There is just less to think about, and this results in the completion of more workouts.

+ Freedom: One of the features I enjoy about my home gym is the freedom that it affords. I can exercise at 2:00 am in the morning if I want to, and can also listen to a radio and watch the TV shows. I can even hog the equipment. I never feel restricted at my home gym.

+ Feeling self-conscious: When you are severely over-weight, it can be intimidating walking into a gym. You may feel as if people are judging you all the time. You may also worry that you might not be using the proper form and technique when lifting, and that people would be commenting on your poor form. When you have all these little things crawling in your mind, it can severely impact your workout. At home, however, I do not have to consider such thoughts.

+ Winter: I have found that it's much easier to get up and workout at home during the winter seasons, especially in the mornings.

+ Taking a break: When taking a break from workouts I am not worried about losing my gym membership fees, or having to freeze my account until I am ready to get back into training. However, I have personally found that it is much easier to get back into my routine when my gym is just next to my bedroom.

Above, I have given some of the reasons for my preference for a home gym. However, those people who love to socialise, enjoy meeting new people, need accessibility to a wide range of equipment and services, and prefer workouts with a 'gym flavor,' should join a public gym.

Having a Training Partner

There is no doubt that exercising with other people can be very beneficial. It can be a great source of motivation and make exercising a more enjoyable routine. However, it also has its drawbacks, something I personally experienced during my Journey.

Let me be blunt. I never enjoyed working with a training partner. The major reason being that you and your training partner may have different needs, requirements, attitudes, levels of motivation and schedules. As a result, you might find it difficult to continually agree on mutual accommodation without your training being negatively impacted. As an example, one of the issues I had with my training partner was that we both had different fitness levels. This resulted in my partner slowing me down. During our workouts, he wanted to head back home after 45 minutes, while I wanted to continue working for another 30. Not only did these types of scenarios caused conflicts, but I always ended up with the feeling that I had not worked out to the best of my ability. On the other hand, if I had trained solo, I would not have been confronted with these issues, and I would have spent my total energy focusing on my goal of working for as long as I wanted and without having to worry about another person standing on queue.

While I have stated that I do not enjoy working with a working/training partner, I do not mean they should be avoided altogether. This is because when you work with a training partner you will show confidence and obtain an accelerated understanding of the values of training and exercises. However, some difficulties may arise if your training partner decides to skip training for one reason or another. This may make you less motivated to exercise and more likely to skip training until he is available the next time. This type of hiatus can be severely detrimental to your weight-loss Journey as it may lead to a loss of momentum, create dependency, and stall your progress.

Based on my own experience, I would highly recommend that you try and get into a habit of training alone. Training alone gives you more control as well as allowing you to work towards your goals without being held back by any other person.

Throw Away Your Scale

If you have a habit of weighing yourself daily on a scale, I highly recommend that you stop using this practice to measure your progress in losing weight because a scale is not a good indicator of how well you are advancing. A faulty reading scale can also have a very demoralising effect on your Journey.

Various unrelated factors determine the number you see on the scale every time you weigh yourself. Personally speaking, small issues like not having a proper bowel movement in the morning usually showed a higher reading on the scale which would cause me to freak out. When I started lifting weights, the scale also indicated that I had put on weight, yet I found myself able to fit into smaller sized clothes. The scale never provided a true reflection of my Journey. Family members who had not seen me for sometime would tell me how much weight I had lost, but the scale indicated that nothing had changed. I am glad I had listened to these independent witnesses rather than depose my faith on the display on the scale. Had I accepted the readings on the scale, I would have given up exercise a long time ago for, as somebody had said "It [the scale] is a poor indicator of progress."

Therefore, do not give a scale the power to influence how you feel, especially when it is not accurate to begin with. If you get rid of the scale, you will be better off without it.

If you want a better method to measure your progress, I have found that the best way to achieve this is to try and fit into a shirt that is too small for you. You will know that you are making progress when the shirt slowly starts to fit. If it gets tighter, you will know that you are putting on weight and that you may need to review your weight loss strategy. This is my approach and it has worked well for me. I would highly suggest that you try this strategy as well.

Make Exercise a Hobby

One of the best ways to commit and stick to your exercise routine is to turn it into a hobby. Instead of treating exercising as an activity which you need to do to lose weight, see if you can make it a pastime that you undertake for leisure and as part of living a healthier lifestyle.

Despite having reached my weight loss goals, I continue taking a huge interest in exercising daily and consuming healthy food, principally vegetables and low-calorie drinks. I still do a lot of reading regularly on walking and weight lifting, and still subscribe to online health communities and forums. I am always looking out for new tips and advice in order to attain self-fulfillment

Nowadays, as part of exercising, I look for new walking tracks and cover as many as I can, and also connect with walking groups and like-minded individuals. For weightlifting, I am always browsing through the internet fora to learn about the best exercises available for building muscles and improving my lifting techniques. I also regularly watch videos to learn how to improve my health and how I can go about trying to reverse the damages I have inflicted on my body.

By taking a keen interest in my health and exercise, I ensure that my enthusiasm for regular exercise is kept at the highest level. I am surprised to experience the enormous joy and happiness that I receive from exercising, especially after I turned it into a hobby. The lifting of weights, walking, cycling, playing cricket in the nets has now become an inalienable part of my life. All these activities help me to recover the body that I once despised and wished to destroy. I would highly encourage that you make your exercise routine not only an activity, but a lifelong hobby. Take serious interest in it, learn as much as you can, and you will be one step closer in ensuring that you live a healthier, fat-free life.

More Ideas to Complement Your Weight Loss Objectives

Usually when people make an undertaking to change, they tend to mistakenly believe that once they have lost weight and achieved their goals, they can revert to their old ways. Regretfully, what they don't realise is that one wrong turn can be the quickest road to regaining the old weight. You should remember that being healthy and staying fit should become a way of life and not an end goal itself.

In the following sections, I will look at additional ideas that will assist you in achieving your weight-loss goals. You should understand that losing weight is not only about diet and exercise; there are a lot of other factors that need to be considered and addressed in order to ensure a successful outcome. The application of a few small changes to your strategy will not only complement your weight loss initiatives but can also lead to a complete life transformation.

Adopting a Minimalistic Lifestyle

One of the biggest changes I made during my Journey was to adopt a minimalistic lifestyle. For those who are not familiar with this concept, a minimalistic lifestyle is the practice of removing all the clutter and noise around so that you live in a simple and modest way. When you have less obligations in life, you will encounter less distractions and thus can focus more of your energy on building what is important in your life. For example, during my struggle with obesity I was focused on achieving weight-loss goals only and nothing else interested me as much. I did not buy unnecessary or expensive consumer items and had made myself comfortable by throwing away or giving things that I did not use to charity. I also did not fill my house with clutters such as little toys, decorations, ornaments, paintings and books. I tried to keep my house as empty as possible and lived a life based on necessity. By keeping my setting in such a manner, I ensured that I maintained a quiet and peaceful environment. The sense of extreme calmness that I felt when I walked into my house had to be experienced to be believable.

Since implementing a minimalistic life, I have freed myself from external interferences and I do not find myself overwhelmed by things that caused me unnecessary worry and stress. In fact, I have yet to miss any items that I had thrown away or chose to forgo. Living frugally has also allowed me to cut down on my living expenses, and I have invested the savings on my health instead; or to purchase goods that are important to me. I will not hesitate to spend good money on a decent pair of walking shoes, on learning a new skill, purchase a musical instrument, or to take up boxing classes. I see all these activities as an investment that will help me grow to become a better and healthy person.

Downsizing my life has been a blessing, especially during the last stages of my Journey. By cultivating a simplistic lifestyle, I have allowed myself not only to enjoy the benefits that come with this lifestyle, but also to truly dedicate all my energy into my weight loss aspirations.

Why the People You Hang Around Matter

The people you surround yourself with will play an important role in your weight-loss journey. If you earnestly want to lose weight and adopt a healthier lifestyle, then you must surround yourself with people who have the same values, vision and goals as yourself. If you are surrounded by people who choose to neglect their health and live an unhealthy lifestyle, then you may find yourself struggling to achieve your weight loss goals. When you associate yourself with non-likeminded people, then it becomes easy to go with the "group flow", and consequently ignoring your own health goals. You should never underestimate the negative influence your peers can have on you, especially if they themselves are overweight and continually tell you that you do not need to lose weight. If you surround yourself with such individuals, then you will make it harder for you to find the motivation you need to undertake needed changes. However, if you surround yourself with like-minded people who are health-conscious and who are interested in their fitness and wellbeing, you will find your transition into your new, healthier lifestyle a lot smoother. If you want to lose weight and live a healthier lifestyle, you must spend time with people who have the same ambitions as you have. When you surround yourself with people who continually encourage you to lose weight, chances are you will try to eliminate all the negative influences that could harm your chances of succeeding.

It will be a good policy if you are not afraid to let go of negative friends whose health values do not align with yours. Have an abundant mentality and realise that new positive friends will enter your life during your change endeavour, to replace the ones you have "fired". If, however, you cannot completely avoid certain people, try to limit your contact with them. Choose wisely those with whom you want to hang around.

Why You Should Forgive People

One of the important parting acts you should perform as part of your transformation is to forgive the people who in the past had hurt you during your Journey. At the risk of being repetitious, obesity can lead a person to experience teasing, bullying, humiliation, loss of self-esteem, depression, feeling of hopelessness, suicidal, and much more. These experiences can cause a person to harbour extreme lifelong hatred and anger towards their tormentors.

When I started my Journey, I was very angry at a lot of people, especially the ones who used to tease me when I was a child. I also had reserved anger towards my parents. I felt as if they had let me down when I was young. I mean, how could they let me become this way? How could they sit there and just watch me go through my life like this? I felt they should have done more, and they certainly should have paid more attention to my health.

However, as I have grown older, I have come to accept that my parents wanted to give me complete control over my life decisions right from an early age. All the factors that contributed to my weight gain occurred because of the decisions I had made, and not anyone else. Now, I accept full culpability for all the traumatic changes that have negatively affected my life at a critical time of my body development. I also understand that my parents were caught up in their own health problems while providing all types of services to me and themselves. With the limited time they had, I feel that they did the best they could with the knowledge they had to help me fight my obesity. Back in the early 90's, there was not much education or awareness about obesity in the public domain in the country of my birth, and support for my parents was minimal. They could not have known how to help me. However, my parents are now retired and have used their time to play an inspirational role in helping me lose weight. I would not have accomplished much without their help and encouragement.

I have also made peace and forgiven all the people who teased and bullied me through my life. I do not hold any hatred or anger towards them anymore, and hope that they have progressed in their lives and have not suffered in any way as I did. As the result of this exoneration, I have managed to free myself from this bugbear of blaming others. If you have bottled within yourself such feelings, see if you can also forgive people who have caused you hurt so as to extricate yourself from all the anger and hate that can unnecessarily increase your blood pressure and engender other medical problems. Such an act of forgiveness may go a long way in ensuring you enjoy your life socially, healthily and spiritually to the fullest.

Developing a Positive Mindset

Developing a positive mindset and outlook towards life will play a crucial role in achieving your weight loss goals. It will ensure that you go through your change process with the right attitude and that you are able to effectively handle the numerous setbacks and impediments that you are likely to encounter during your Journey.

In order to develop a positive mindset, the first thing you must do is to efface from your memory the vestiges of the past, like releasing the pressure from a cylinder full of gas. Once this happens, your mind becomes devoid of those past images. They will no longer exist. Therefore, it is pointless holding on to them any longer. Make peace with them, and let them disappear from your body. I fully understand why you might still be angry at others for treating you badly when you were growing up. I understand your deep hurt, as I was also ridiculed constantly over my obese situation while having no choice but had to go on with my life every day and face the ridicule and humiliation over and over. But I have no doubt that with experience and wisdom gained over the passage of time you will become a stronger and a forethoughtful person.

One thing you must not forget is that no amount of your anger will change the past. Anger will always remain in the present, set in stone. It becomes past once eliminated. Your present is your Journey and you must make peace with whatever anger you have to successfully complete your weight reduction objectives. Only a peaceful mind can facilitate your struggle, while a chaotic and a confused mind is likely to derail you from your chosen path. You must learn to exploit your negative and painful past experiences as life lessons and use them to change your current situation for your personal resurrection and regeneration.

Another regret, as hard as it may be to accept, is that you must also come to terms with the fact that while fighting obesity, you had missed out on significant parts of your enjoyable life which cannot be duplicated, such as your teenage years. For example, I find it painful to remember at having missed out on socialisation and dating in my teens and twenties because my obesity limited these opportunities. Once out of the doldrums, I had to rebuild my social skills and become comfortable around women. All these social interruptions had a detrimental psychological impact on me later in life. However, now I accept the inevitability of just how things turned out in my life and look forward to enjoying all the new adventures in my 30s, as it is never too late to enjoy a life of total fulfilment.

If you are reading this book, you must now make a promise that from now on you will take full responsibility of your body and health, and that you will choose not to dwell in the past anymore. You must accept that certain precious pieces of your life have gone forever and that there are still a lot of opportunities for you to enjoy in the future years.

Finally, you must show compassion and kindness to people around you. You should want to become the person who, despite being on the wrong end of life, still has the heart and strength to show kindness to people. You must not remain bitter or angry. How many people are there in this world who are bitter because their lives did not turn out the way they expected? How many people do you know who want others to suffer because they suffered themselves? You do not want to be this person. You are better than them. Your values are higher than theirs.

So, develop a positive mindset today. Let go of the past, and help yourself and the world. By having a positive approach, you will make a positive impact in nourishing and sustaining your renovated body.

Give Up Alcohol and Cigarettes

The abstention of alcohol and cigarettes permanently from your daily menu should be an integral part of your weight loss endeavour. These two items add no value whatsoever to your body and health in general. If anything, they will make your wallet lighter, create many health problems and hinder your ability to complete your weight loss transformation in a timely manner.

In my case, aside from many health issues related to alcohol and cigarettes, the main reason I gave up these vices was that they significantly contributed to the occurrence of relapse. On a few occasions, I had succumbed to the temptation of buying a packet of cigarettes which had resulted in months of binge eating. Just a single packet! I had even experienced undoing months of progress just by participating in one drinking session. It is not just the drinking session that caused the problem; it is what happened the following morning. Not only was I hung over and unable to exercise, but more detrimentally I craved for sugar and binged on sugary foods. I found it difficult to resist these foods and binged for a few weeks before steadying myself and continued with my Journey. While some individuals may be able to incorporate alcohol and cigarettes into their lifestyle without any ill effects, I had found that these two items were huge impediments. I addressed this problem, with great difficulty, by removing these two items completely from my life. For these reasons, I advise you to keep these two 'noxious' stuffs away from your body.

Socialisation

One of the biggest problems I faced during my Journey related to socialisation. After making significant improvement in reducing my weight, I found it difficult to commence socialising without sacrificing the gains achieved thus far. I found myself in an imbroglio.

Most of my friends and family members loved drinking and

eating rich meals. However, I had removed these items from my diet as part of my weight loss strategy. I did not find any fun in participating in these events so I invariably avoided them thereby increasing my feelings of alienation and loneliness. The alternative was to go to a restaurant for a small meal, meet somebody and start a conversation. However, the fear I had was the potential of a 'small meal' turning into a 'big meal' mixed with an unlimited consumption of alcohol and falling into a relapse. So, in order to avoid this trap, I would usually take Chinese tea, few tomatoes, fruits such as apple, banana, and boiled eggs, followed by a walk with few of my close friends and family members. Instead of having a big alcohol-fueled night out and eating food at restaurants, or buying coffee daily, I preferred walking instead. I found this to be a healthier alternative. Not only was I furthering my own goals, but I was also helping my family and friends into exercising. It was a win-win situation. Furthermore, if ever I found myself at a social gathering where alcohol and sugary items were being served, I would instead request a cup of tea with no sugar or just drink a glass of water. I also made sure that I did not succumb to peer pressure in these situations.

To ensure a permanent result, I took time to phase out my previous unhealthy habits. I made it a habit to tell all the new people I met that I did not drink alcohol or smoke, and casually told them about my new lifestyle. I never mentioned to them that I was trying to lose weight or that I used to drink and smoke. This ensured that all the new people that came into my life knew about my preferences, saw me as a person who did not drink alcohol or smoke, and as a result never asked me out for drinks or offered me a cigarette.

To the existing people who were aware of my past habits, I told them that I was growing bored of drinking, smoking and eating fast food, and that I was more interested in my health.

Initially there was some resistance, but eventually they got the hint. Believe me, I was also happy to ditch them if they were not supportive of my lifestyle changes, but luckily, I never had to go down that path.

You must remember that some people in your life will move out and new ones will come in. One day you may be surprised to find that you are surrounded by a completely new set of people and they would only know you by your new lifestyle, not by your old one. If you phase out your bad habits, socialising would become much easier.

Use Your Journey to Inspire Others

While undertaking your weight-loss transformation, you should also take the opportunity to inspire and help other people who might be in the same boat as you are on. The experience and knowledge that you accumulate during your own Journey might be invaluable to other people about to begin or who are already on their weight loss plan. You should take this opportunity not only to become a role model to others, but also a voice and expert that gives people hope and an inspiration to lose weight.

While I was still on my Journey, I posted 30 second video clips of all the food that I ate during the day on my social media accounts. It was like a food video blog. Initially, I did this for fun but soon realised that a large number of people had started to take interest in my progress by following my accounts. This resulted in a significant boost to my confidence and motivational levels as I could see myself inspiring others to adopt and change their lifestyle.

If you are game enough, take before and after pictures of yourself. Document your progress and post your results and success on health community fora and social media. Lead the way and show people what can be achieved. This will not only inspire others but will give you the drive you need to push yourself even further. If you do not want to take your story online, then you should instead try to inspire your family members and friends to adopt a healthier lifestyle. Show them how much your life has improved and encourage them to emulate you. By inspiring others to lose weight, you will be pushing yourself further into permanently committing to your new lifestyle, and you may never know who will be watching your progress. You may be surprised at the opportunities that open when people observe the positive impact you are having on others. So, go out there and inspire people!

Gamification

If you have done enough research on losing weight, I have no doubt you would have come across numerous articles that claim that a diet overhaul, daily exercise and a significant lifestyle change are the major ingredients needed to achieve a permanent weight loss. I have no doubt in my mind that a lot of individuals who have already lost weight, either partially or permanently, would have focused on these elements. However, for an individual like me, who had continuously failed in all previous attempts to lose weight despite addressing the three key factors, the application of the gamification strategies gave me the ability to achieve my goals and boosted my strength. I have no hesitation in claiming that gamification had played a critical role in my personal transformation, and is perhaps one of the main reasons for my success. It had been the driving factor that allowed me to overcome past failures and to continue pushing my boundaries.

Through gamification techniques I had turned my weight loss Journey into a highly addictive game.

When I initially kicked off my Journey, I was filled with excitement. I envisioned a future full of opportunities. I enjoyed getting up every morning and looked forward with enthusiasm to exercise and to eat healthy food. However, as weeks went on, my enthusiasm and motivational levels declined, and then I went into several incidents of relapse. However, I am not the type of person who gives up on things easily, so I repeated the entire process with the aid of gamification and then quickly found myself walking down the familiar path towards recovery. During this period of the adoption of additional approaches to weight loss initiatives, I played an imaginary game which required alignment of gamification activities to my strengths. The results were unbelievable, and this simple gamely experiment immediately captured my thoughts. This is how I got infatuated with the concept. It boosted my creativity, improved my communication and imaginative skills and put me back on the road to the rejuvenation of my body.

The Art of Gaming

In this section, I would like to discuss the reasons that led me to apply the concept of gaming techniques as a panacea for my weight burden. It all started a couple of years ago when I had started working as a computer consultant for a small IT firm. The work was decent, but there was one aspect of the job that I did not enjoy a bit — it was the daily commute. It took me an hour and a half to get to work daily, and I felt that the entire journey was too long and boring. To help pass time, I started playing games such as 'Temple Run' and 'Subway Surfers' on my mobile phone. If you have never heard or played these games, all I would like to convey is that they can be very addictive, and I played these games non-stop for months on my train journeys. Eventually, I wondered what were the secrets of my addiction to these games? What instantly attracted me to these games once I was on the train? But I did not personally find anything captivating about these games as they involved just running about — that's it, just running and running until you got caught by a person or creature chasing you. On paper, it was just a boring repetitive game. Then why was I playing the games so often? After careful examination, I learnt that what really drew me to these games over and over were their objectives and missions. I found them interesting and quite challenging. There was a high level of motivation from my side to complete all the missions that the developers had created for their games, and if I did not complete a mission with a perfect score, I would be required to repeat the missions until I achieved the perfect objective. All these led me to suddenly ask a few questions. What if I created a game of this nature to address my weight loss objectives? — a game that could be built upon the concepts and ideas of gamification and on my strengths. What if I could replicate the addictive nature of these games and then apply them to my own weight loss objectives? I asked. It was at this stage when several ideas germinated in my mind as to how to add gamely elements into my weight loss strategies. Later, once these thoughts had crystallised, I applied the gamification concept to my weight loss plan.

Losing Weight Through Gamification

As I have a background in information technology, I was able to create gamification activities in an Excel spreadsheet (See Table

2). It had no graphics or audio and was simple and minimalistic in design. The game did require manual inputting of data, but certain cells were automatically calculated. The objective of this game was to enable me to eliminate all the negative influences in my life that were preventing me from attaining self-fulfilment. Let me explain the nature of this game with an example. Suppose I played these games from 1st May 2015 to 31st December 2015, as shown in Columns B and C (see Table 2). The ultimate purpose and goal of playing this game was to help me cut down on food items that were contributing to my weight gain. However, there was a limit to what diet, exercising and lifestyle changes could do to help me achieve my weight-reduction goals, as there were incidence of relapse and recovery after months of binge eating. But by incorporating games into my Journey I was able to control my sugar binge, avoid food that increased my weight, and received tremendous boost in confidence to accelerate completion of my weight loss objectives. In playing these games, I created some interesting objectives for myself. These missions were heavily influenced by the game 'Temple Run' which I played on my IPhone. Some examples of these missions included:

+ Score 25,000 points
+ Collect 500 coins
+ Run 1000m without collecting a coin.

Table 2: My games based on Gamification

	A	B	C	D	E	F	G	H	I
1	Cutting Down	Start Date	Today Date	Days Overall Success	Current Success Streak	Fail	Previous Attempt %	Success %	High Score
2	Biscuit	1/05/15	31/12/15	223		21		91%	
3	Smoking	1/05/15	31/12/15	227		17		93%	
4	Chocolate	1/05/15	31/12/15	227		17		93%	
5	Sugar	1/05/5	31/12/15	227		17		93%	
6	Bread & Margarine	1/05/15	31/12/15	233		11		95%	
7	Coffee & Milo	1/05/15	31/12/15	236		8		97%	
8	Milk	1/05/15	31/12/15	233		11		95%	
9	Pastries (Cake, Donut)	1/05/15	31/12/15	227		17		93%	
10	Wine	1/05/15	31/12/15	241		3		99%	
11	Bread (Excluding Wholemeal)	1/05/15	31/12/15	238		6		98%	
12	Prescription Drugs (Excluding CD)	1/05/15	31/12/15	244				100%	
13	Flu	1/05/15	31/12/15	244				100%	
14	Fast Food	1/05/15	31/12/15	244				100%	
15	Cereal (Excluding Wheat Biscuits)	1/05/15	31/12/15	244				100%	
16	Alcohol	1/05/15	31/12/15	242		2		99%	
17	Ice Cream	1/05/15	31/12/15	241		3		99%	
18	Soft Drinks (Coke, Soda, etc)	1/05/15	31/12/15	242		2		99%	
19	Retail Soap	1/05/15	31/12/15	244				100%	
20	Retail Shampoo	1/05/15	31/12/15	244				100%	
21	Deodorant	1/05/15	31/12/15	241		3		99%	
22	Potato Chips	1/05/15	31/12/15	242		2		99%	
23	Restaurant Food	1/05/15	31/12/15	244				100%	
24	Artificial Sweetners	1/05/15	31/12/15	244				100%	

Table 3: Column Definitions for the Gamification score

Column	Name	Definition
A	Cutting Down	I wrote down a list of all the negative influences in my life that were contributing to my weight gain. These included items such as sugar, biscuits, and pastries. As my goal was not only to lose weight and become healthier, but to change my entire life around, I reduced related items such as smoking, consuming alcohol and prescription medication (unless it was absolutely required).
B	Start Date	This is the date I decided that I would start abstaining from all the items listed in **Column A.**
C	Today's Date	A column which listed the current date, used for calculations.
D	Overall Success Days	This is the **overall** number of days that I had managed to go without the items I had listed in Column A. **Calculation: Column B — Column F**
E	Current Success Streak	The number of days I had managed to abstain from consuming the items in my list since a FAIL. **Calculation: Column C — Column G**
F	Fail	If I ended up consuming an item on my list on a particular day it would count as a fail, and 1 would be added to this column instead of being added to Column D. This eventually would become the total number of days I consumed an item during my game.
G	Streak Start Date	After a fail, I would add the following days date to restart my streak.
H	Success Column	Showed a percentage of how many days I had managed to refrain from the items on my list.
I	High Score	This showed the highest number of days I had gone without a fail during a streak. If I had a fail, I would add the number of days I had gone without an item as my high score. This would become the score I would try to beat in my next streak

Using the above examples, I then created similar missions for myself. Some examples of these included:

+ Ensure Success is maintained at 95% for all items listed;
+ Do not drink alcohol or smoke cigarettes for 60 days; and
+ Ensure that you do not fail more than three times on all the items listed.

I had created these types of challenges for over a period of two years. When I started to play these games, I failed miserably. I was not able to accomplish any of the missions that I had established and easily surrendered. However, I did realise at that time that regular practice was the key to success, and acting on this realisation I became better at completing my missions. The first game that I successfully completed lasted a week. Eventually I played a game that lasted an entire year. Even though it could not be regarded as a perfect game, the results showed that I had lost weight. My happiness knew no bounds!

The Results

After experiencing success and having played the game for a while, I felt assured that I could achieve any goal and became prepared to face any future challenge. I had garnered so much courage and thus had no intention to run away any more from my problems, or to use food as a source of comfort. Upon completing a game each time, I also gained more insight on problems that were of major concern to me. From the games that I played, I found that smoking, eating biscuits and pastries were matters of serious concern. However, soft drinks, potato chips and alcohol were not. This information was crucial as it allowed me to target the problematic areas that were impeding my Journey. One thing you must remember is that the games I played were relatively simple and completely flexible. I had set my own rules and objectives. However, with this flexibility came the option to cheat and to make exceptions. Notwithstanding, if there was one important lesson that I had learnt from playing these games, it was the value of complete honesty and how to accept and overcome disappointments. After playing these games and scrutinising the results, I removed a number of unhealthy foods from my diet, foods that I previously thought I needed and could not live without. By adding the technique of *gamification* to my plan, I had lost a lot of weight as well as improved my chances of permanently keeping it under control. This game-show later became one of the most important tools in reducing my weight.

The Power of Success and a High Score

There are two columns in this game, as shown in Table 3. These are the SUCCESS and HIGH SCORE. As I gradually showed more skills at playing these games, I started to gain success days and high scores. Each time I was tempted by food the first thing that flashed into my mind was high score. I also noted that the higher my score went, the more energy I needed in maintaining my record. In this way, I went through many months without all the unhealthy items on my list, which directly resulted in accelerating my Journey to the end. Gamification had not only given me the opportunity to learn about myself but also enabled me to feel myself healthier every day and be totally in control of my body.

Now, I would want you to start thinking about creating something — a game or an idea — that would complement your dieting and exercising efforts and challenge you to lead a life of fulfilment. If you are able to integrate such an idea or game into your personality strengths and then analyse the results, I have no doubt in my mind that you would feel how beautiful life is and why you should fight for it.

Setting a Realistic Timeframe to Lose Weight

It is very common for people to incorrectly estimate the length of time that should elapse before noticing a significant loss of weight. They always take the mistaken view that their entire weight loss steps would take less than the realistic time. However, as I learnt later to my bitter disappointment, this conclusion is a bit stupid as it is extremely difficult for a person to reverse an unhealthy and chaotic lifestyle in a fixed time. That is why setting a realistic timeframe at the inchoate phase of the Journey is extremely important. People who set unrealistic timeframes feel demoralised and depressed when their expectations are not met within that timeframe, and may eventually give up the struggle. Therefore, you must jettison the notion from your mind that years of unhealthy and undesirable living can be reversed in a few months or years. This is simply not possible, as burning body fat is a much more difficult task than cutting down weight. If you do not believe in this assessment, then not only are you making your goals harder to achieve but you are declaring that you lack the mental strength to succeed, and thus all further attempts are likely to culminate in failure. It took me over two years to reverse almost over twenty years of living an unhealthy, humiliating, depressive, suicidal and deplorable life. If you do not observe or feel you have lost weight within a realistic timeframe, then it could be an indication that you have not assiduously followed a credible weight loss plan. In any case, I must admit that a successful loss weight plan will depend upon a range of diverse factors, because overweight bodies are composed of different building materials or genes and their demolition to a desirable size will take a lot more time.

Finally, the setting of a realistic timeframe to achieve your weight loss goals cannot be over-emphasised. An unrealistic time frame will stymie your progress towards your desired destination and it is for this reason that a regular and rigorous scrutiny and adjustment of your weight loss plan is essential at different stages of your Journey. As Robbins (1991) warned: "If you raise your standards but don't really believe you can meet them, you've already sabotaged yourself."(p.24)

Telling People that You are Trying to Lose Weight

Previously, I had discussed that after you have successfully overcome your weighty problem, you should inspire and motivate the people around you to lose weight and adopt a healthier lifestyle. Whether you are a tutor or a student or both, there are certain factors you should consider such as disclosure of personal information, especially if you plan to share your weight loss goals, aspirations and success with the people around you.

The reason I have brought the issue of revealing personal information is because once you disclose your intention to others, you will find that there will be a few people around you who will discourage you to lose weight and secretly want you to fail. These types of saboteurs do exist.

You must remember that a person who has lost weight becomes a symbol of success and that success breeds hate and jealousy. Without you realising it, there is a chance that your weight loss could make the people hovering around you to feel inadequate and inferior, and consequently these people will project feelings of dislike and resentment towards you. The more progress you make, the more they will feel that you do not deserve downsizing. If you browse across the social media and the internet sites on the topics relating to obesity and weight loss issues, you will find that a lot of readers direct hateful and humiliating comments towards people who have successfully fought obesity. Look at the websites of celebrities and prominent people and read the spiteful and humiliating comments about them.

When you decide to participate in a weight loss marathon, there should be no doubt in your mind about your objective, which is to reduce your weight. For taking this initiative, you can expect feelings of hatred from some people in your own circle. Never pretend that these types of people don't exist when they do. Remember that their own inability to improve their current situation is causing them to inflict anger towards people who, through tremendous personal sacrifice and determination, are trying to do something to stabilise their health. These people cannot see themselves getting anywhere in life, so they want others to stay with them. The best way to deal with these phenomena is to observe the key signs of their frustration and not to allow them and their toxic hatred and jealousy to stop you from achieving your goals. However, once you have successfully reached your destination, you may decide to show resilience and compassion when interacting with such people. You should find a way to tolerate their hatred and at the same time ensure that it does not affect you personally or your ambitions. At worst, there is no harm in ditching them, especially if you feel that they will continue to sabotage your personal plans.

During your Journey, it will be a good policy to remain humble and say less than the requirement. If needed, share your Journey with supportive people like your family and close friends — people you trust and know won't feel threatened. The rest of the world does not need to know what you are getting up to. However, if you are comfortable feel free to inspire everyone using your experience. Never boast and always help the people around you to achieve their own goals. However, do not waste your time on haters; instead use that time to consolidate your own achievements. Finally, something that I had learnt from my Journey: the more hatred and jealousy is directed at you means the better you are doing.

Weight-Loss Advertising and Marketing

There is a wealth of information available to us on diets, health and exercises on the internet. All the information and the products we need, ranging from solid nutritional advice to weight management tips, are just a few clicks away.

However, an important point to remember is that while there are genuine products and services available in the market putatively fighting obesity, they often have to compete with fake products and services that are commercial in orientation. In my opinion, the weight-loss industry is full of lies, deception and manipulation and we must use discretion when buying their products.

Many large businesses use a variety of methods and techniques to determine the best way to make money out of 'confused' people facing a wide range of health issues. They will often use highly specialised marketing campaigns to convince innocent people like you and me to buy trivial things that are not effective in fighting obesity. During my Journey, I had spent a lot of time and money in trying out various diets, blindly followed internet advice and frequently bought several products including weight loss supplements. Only a few of them were of help to me, the rest were spurious.

Should you ever find yourself caught up in these sinister moments, make sure that you are not fooled by the information that comes with the products and services that make exaggerated claims or give over the top promises. Such messages are usually designed to take advantage of the desperate and vulnerable people. This is where self-education becomes important. Ensure that you always do adequate research and make decisions based on genuine information. Do not ever blindly follow or believe what you read or hear. This means you must carry out a thorough homework before making a purchase.

However, the most important thing to remember is that you should not spend too much time getting caught up with all the weight loss advertising and marketing fluff around you. You do not need 99% of the weight-loss panacea sold in the open market and you can still reach your desired destination without using them.

Finalising Your Weight-Loss Strategy and Action.

If you are prepared and ready to start your maiden Journey, then it is now time to walk the talk. This stage is probably one of the most important segments of your weighty plan. Imagine that you are at the bottom of a mountain and you have started to climb it. You must not show any fear to undertake the first step; if you do, then you may be considered inadequate physically and psychologically to complete this marathon. In my personal experience, this was one of the most satisfying activities in my life. Once I had covered half the Journey, I felt as if I had matured more and being transformed into a superman. I also felt unafraid to take the remaining steps to the top, an objective I initially thought would be beyond my physical endurance.

In the previous sections, I had discussed important ideas,

tactics and strategies that could be used to plan and formulate weight loss strategies.

To begin with, at the action stage you should have a weight loss plan in place, or at least have an idea as to what steps you will need to take to achieve your weight loss goals. If you don't have this, then it is not too late to formulate one, which will need regular refinement once you have started your Journey. As I had explained in previous sections of this book, my plan consisted of a simple custom diet that was very low in sugar, weight lifting, walking, and the application of gamification technique. This technique involved the creation of two spreadsheets to track my weight lifting scores and what negative influences to avoid. So, this was my weight loss plan. Very simple indeed. Remember, a plan can be a very simple one, or a very complex one. There can be all types of variations in between these two extremes.

Once you have completed your Journey, what happens next? Well, you should not sit down on your laurels and start singing that "it is all over" or "I have survived." No, the Journey is not over, not yet. If you go back to your previous indulgences, you will be deliberately sabotaging your health. Is this what you want after months and years of weighty marathons? Most probably not. If I heard you correctly, then you must prepare a plan that you should implement to sustain your weight at least at the current level. If you read the plan that I had crafted and implemented, you will easily understand what message I am trying to convey.

Having Trouble Getting Started

Getting started can be difficult for some people as it takes a lot of effort and energy. As a result, they end up simply procrastinating. However, as I have learnt when I decided to participate in my Journey, time moves fast — in fact, real fast. If you lose your weight drastically, your entire life can change for the better, and unlike me, you do not want to be that guy who wished he had taken action sooner. That is why it is important that you start acting on your weight loss plan immediately. Do not delay, and make achieving your weight loss goals one of your life's highest priorities. In my opinion, the best way to get the ball rolling is by starting off small. If your weight loss plan is superfluous and unsustainable in the long run, make it simpler by trimming it down. However, if you are continually struggling to get started despite making your plan simpler, I would advise you to create a very basic action plan and make an effort to maintain it for six weeks. During this six week routine, you can gradually start cutting out unhealthy foods from your diet and undertake thirty minutes of exercise three times a week. I am trying to keep it very simple at the moment. Understand that everything does not need to happen all at once, and that your weight loss plan can be built over a period of time. It is perfectly acceptable to slowly transition into your new lifestyle.

Another important point to remember is that you should not distract yourself from taking real action by spending time reading and researching about health. You may be under the impression that you are working towards your goals by gaining all this knowledge, but it will not help you lose weight unless you convert it into action. In any case, there is a limit to how much a person can read and research. If you keep on gluing yourself to these distractions once you have "mounted the horse", they just become a form of procrastination. It is only by getting into action and sweating that you will you be able to get the ball rolling and achieve some or all your objectives in one session.

As a matter of fact, the starting point is the toughest and the most unnerving phase but, as I said before, until you start rolling the ball you will not be able to see the light at the end of the tunnel. However, if your nerves stop you from starting, then unfortunately you have to force yourself into action. I have quite often heard that fear is the greatest enemy of success, so do not let fear drag you into lethargy and inaction. The overwhelming reason for your wish to reduce weight is to regain your health and self-esteem. Remember that you always wanted to lose weight, and once you get going you will wish that you had started sooner.

The Point of No Return

Let me assume that you have successfully written a weight loss plan and that you have rolled the ball. Now visualise your Journey as a steep mountain climb. You will start your Journey at the bottom and your goal and objectives are to reach to the top. While the ultimate goal is to reach the top, your initial objective will be to reach the "Point of No Return" (PNR). (See Figure 5)

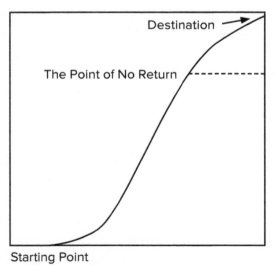

Figure 5: The Point of No Return (PNR)

The PNR is a specific moment in your Journey where continuation up the mountain outweighs the benefits of returning all the way down. This is where you might say to yourself, "I am enjoying life right now as a result of this climb" or "I just cannot afford to go back down anymore, since I have climbed up too far". Those who reach the PNR truly experience measurable results, such as reduction in weight and enhance their skills in food management. Furthermore, they discover that their self-worth and confidence have risen to an all-time high. People around them compliment them about their appearance and reach out to them for weight loss advice and tips. They also suddenly find themselves becoming a role model for others and see life from a different perspective. This only motivates them to climb higher and higher as they realise that there are more rewards and opportunities by completing their Journey.

Even though the end of the Journey may still be far away at this point, I had found that 'climbing' up to the PNR per se to be a prodigious achievement. It was an exhilarating experience for me to truly feel that by successfully implementing my plan to the very end, I had regained my self-control and the path to self-mastery. It was also a poignant moment when I firmly decided never ever to return to my former self. One important piece of advice that I would like to give is that reaching the PNR becomes your first objective in your Journey. Once you have reached this point, you are deemed to have achieved partial victory and it will also give you a huge psychological boost to complete the Journey.

After reaching the PNR you should feel proud of your decision to reduce your weight, and any doubt about completing the Journey would evaporate. More importantly, once you reach this point, your new habits will become permanent and you should practically be on cruise control for the remainder of the climb.

Building Momentum

In the previous section, I compared your weight loss programme to that of climbing a steep mountain in which the further you progressed, the harder you would expect the ascent to become. One of the key factors that will ensure you are able to successfully reach the top of the mountain is your ability to build and maintain momentum. Greater momentum will provide you with the drive and energy required to successfully reach the top. It is an important force that must be utilised in your plan.

Momentum can be pictured as a snowball being pushed down a hill. As the snowball rolls, it accumulates additional snow, becoming larger and more powerful in the process, until it eventually becomes an unstoppable force. However, the snowball cannot start rolling down the hill unless it is pushed, and this part can be very difficult for some people. Should a push not occur in a timely manner, the snowball will remain on the top of the mountain and will find itself growing smaller and smaller until it is no more. Now I want you to picture that snowball being you. If you are struggling to build momentum, you must remember that all it takes is a small push to get started, and this push needs to happen if you are to succeed. However, remember that once you get the ball rolling, you will encounter obstacles and roadblocks during your downhill roll. These obstacles have the possibility to bring your momentum to a complete halt. Change of jobs, travelling, sickness, family commitments, amongst other factors, are all examples of momentum killers. However, you should expect that your momentum will take numerous hits during your Journey. You must be ready to handle these obstacles as they appear.

During my Journey, I had lost momentum on several occasions. Whenever I lost my momentum, I turned my focus to exercising. This involved taking a ten-minute walk or completing a 2-set workout. These small activities all contributed to a successful resurrection and continuation of my Journey. However, there were certain times when I had to use sheer force, determination and willpower to get moving. These personal attributes were the only ones I needed to gain momentum. These small actions might seem very small and insignificant to a few people; however, they were sufficient to get the snowball rolling. With the passage of each day, I slowly and gradually gained more momentum. I realised that if I did not make it through the initial phase, I would fall back by 6-8 days. The same principle was also applied to my diet. I knew that if I could stick to my healthy eating for a week, I would continue to do so in the weeks ahead. However, here is my single best tip to help you build momentum: Go into your workout with the intention of finishing up in fifteen minutes. You should do this no matter how bad you feel. You will find, more often than not, that after fifteen minutes, you will be heading towards a full, complete workout. I usually went into my workouts with the intention of finishing by 3 sets, however I ended up usually completing my entire routine. I hope you now can appreciate and realise the importance of momentum in exercising. Possessing full momentum should be an absolute must. It will ensure that you are moving forward instead of being stuck.

Make Your First Attempt Count

As soon as you operationalise your weight-loss plan, you must make a personal pledge that you will successfully implement all the stages of your plan. When I started my Journey, I woke up at 5am in the morning during winter and then completed a thorough workout. I walked on the treadmill for an hour daily without getting bored. I followed my workout plan religiously and obtained some of my best results during this period. This was my first and best initial attempt. However, on a few occasions I fell into a relapse and consequently lost all the progress I had made, and then had spent a few long months making half-hearted attempts to resume my Journey. After a few years, when I had finally fig-ured things out and started taking my weight loss plan more seri-ously, I felt that there were a lot of changes in my body and mind. I was not the same person anymore. Age appeared to be playing its proper role.

Below is a list of changes I had experienced when I imple-mented my weight-loss plan seriously:

+ I suddenly found myself unable to walk on the tread mill for more than 20 minutes. I was bored now;
+ I was not making solid muscle gains as quickly as I did previously. It was taking me longer to recover from my workouts as well;
+ I was losing weight a lot slowly;
+ I was struggling to complete walking on the street with my bag with heavy weights;
+ I was not as excited or enthusiastic about the future; and
+ I was starting to feel that it was too late to join the Journey and that even if I did accomplish my goals, I would be too old to enjoy what I would accomplish.

You may now be curious to know the importance of the above observations.

Well, the point I am trying to make here is that it is very important to make your weight loss effort count as early as you can. As I had discovered during my mission, every time I relapsed and quit my subsequent attempts did not have the same passion, motivation and drive as my previous attempts. Every time I came back, my weight loss goals seemed harder to accomplish, and the inner drive I possessed initially had emasculated.

I have learnt that as the body ages, significant life events occur that are capable of changing your personality forever. The opportunities you have today for achieving the major goals of life may not be present in the future. When you first start working on your weight loss goal, you will be replete with enthusiasm and energy. So, make this count and use it to succeed, as every time you fall into a relapse, you end up losing a bit of your initial spirit, and recouping the initial momentum just becomes a bit harder.

My advice to you is to stick to your weight loss strategy, even if you go into a relapse. Never give up, or go backwards and ensure that you make your first effort count. Keep in mind that this is the last time you are going to start to lose weight. After this initial foray, it will be all about maintaining it.

Motivating Yourself

You will be full of enthusiasm and motivation during the initial stages of your weight loss endeavour. The excitement of undertaking your new Journey will ensure that all your efforts and energy are utilised into your routine. However, given the long nature of achieving your ultimate goal, it is usually common to notice a decline in efforts and motivational levels once the initial high enthusiasm wears off, and other life priorities start knocking on the door. For the most part, this decline in motivational levels is expected and should be reversed.

A variety of reasons may have caused a decline in your motivational levels. These include:
+ You are not seeing the results that you are after;
+ You start feeling that losing weight is not achievable;
+ You underestimated the time that it would take to lose weight;

- You are starting to feel that your weight loss plan can wait;
- Your life circumstances have changed and you have other higher priorities as a result;
- You find that people are not responding to you in the way you want them to, thus becoming demotivated; and finally
- You have burnt yourself out.

All the observations mentioned above are momentum killers and are legitimate reasons as to why a person can lose motivation. However, you must remember that unless you stick to our weight loss plan for a significant period of time, success will become elusive.

During the times when motivational levels are low, you must constantly remind yourself as to why you had decided to participate in this activity in the first place. You must close your eyes and visualise all the good things you look forward to experience once you successfully achieve your goal.

When I struggled with the issues related to motivation, I reminded myself that by strictly sticking to my plan even during troubled times, was what a potential winner should emulate. All participants, despite how they feel during their activities, should never allow low levels of motivation stopping them from tasting victory. It has been written that muscles are built during resting periods, and not during weight lifting. Similarly, I do believe that success is not achieved during your best days, but during times when you feel like giving up but still drag on.

One of the best pieces of advice that I had received on motivation was from a work colleague who said that our brain will give you 100 reasons to give up or slack off, but you must stick to your plan regardless of your brain's interference. Even after a big night out, you must wake up the next day and remain action-oriented. This is the level of dedication and commitment that is needed for success and you must take personal responsibility to sustain your motivational levels at all times. However, a certain amount of loss of motivation would be inevitable during your struggle with obesity, and you yourself have to find the right balance with which to maintain your motivational level to achieve progress. Use pure force, if necessary, to get through these low periods, but never give up or display laxity.

Using Small Achievements as Motivation

The small achievements that you make during your 'march' will play an important role in maintaining your momentum and push you to move forward. Every time you accomplish a part of your goal, it is very important to celebrate your success.

Despite several setbacks, I had accomplished a lot during my weight loss mission, and it were these minor accomplishments that generated the necessary motivation to move forward and avoid relapse.

Some of my achievements during my Journey included:

+ Developing the ability to say 'No' to junk food;
+ Overcoming sugar addiction;
+ The ability to stand around smokers without having the urge to smoke;
+ Going 90 days without binge eating;
+ Not catching the flu or taking any medicines for an entire year;
+ Going from shirt size 3XL to a smaller size; and
+ Progressing to deadlift at 100 kilos.

My greatest minor achievement was my ability to carry out a single push-up. Previously, I had never succeeded at this aspect of exercising. This was a momentous occasion and a life changer. Now I can repeat the same exercise without any difficulty. So, always give yourself credit for your accomplishments, no matter how small. It will go a long way in opening your mind as to what is possible, and to provide you with the motivation to push yourself even further and exploit other opportunities.

Symptoms of the Healing Process

I have already discussed in detail about how joining and completing the weight loss Journey can be a hugely challenging assignment. However, once action has been taken, your body will undergo a series of changes as it slowly begins to adjust to your new lifestyle. If you have made significant changes to your diet by introducing healthier food into your system, then you may experience the symptoms of body detoxification. This can be an unpleasant experience for some individuals, as it tends to take the body through the withdrawal process and then removes toxins that have accumulated in the body. During my struggle, I also experienced a variety of symptoms associated with detoxification. It happened when I discarded all junk food from my diet and replaced it with fruits, vegetables and regular exercising.

Below is a list of symptoms that I experienced due to detoxification:

+ Extreme tiredness;
+ Body aches and pains;
+ Hair loss;
+ Blurry vision;
+ Loss in productivity;
+ Constantly becoming sick;
+ Unpredictable sleeping patterns;
+ Irritability and moodiness;
+ Easily angered;
+ Sores and itchiness on skin; and

+ Depression and perpetual sadness.

These symptoms are not constant and can vary from person to person. The good news is that they are only of a temporary nature and should disappear over time.

Managing the Symptoms of Detoxification

During my Journey, I frequently faced all or some symptoms of detoxification at different intervals. I thought I was going cold turkey and had one hell of an experience. I still remember that at one point I had become so aggressive that all I wanted to do was to strangle anyone who came close to me.

These symptoms were not easy to manage, especially when I had to mix work with my university study. But no matter how bad it got, I treated these symptoms as temporary, and luckily, I sailed through them. However, I found that the duration of some of these symptoms lasted much longer than I had expected. But, given the considerable amount of years I had lived an unhealthy life, I consoled myself by muttering that this was fair enough.

Should you experience severe detoxification symptoms, I would like to offer you a few tips to get through them:

+ Understand that overcoming this experience will only make you stronger as a person, and lead to better life opportunities;
+ Inform the people around you of what is happening, so that they understand and can be more supportive towards you;
+ Understand that these symptoms are temporary and eventually they will subside;
+ Undertake exercising to help ease the removal of toxins;

+ Ensure that you drink at least a litre of water every day;
+ Sip warm lemon water throughout the day. I drank a generous amount of Rooibos tea;
+ Make sure that you keep the bowels moving;
+ Use this as an opportunity to learn, and share your experience with others; and
+ Ensure you remain positive throughout the entire experience.

Please never forget that your body is healing itself after so many years of living an unhealthy lifestyle. It is repairing the damage that you have incurred due to neglect. These damages are not permanent and will eventually go away. You must do everything possible to keep on nourishing your body and complete the process of total recovery.

How Do I Socialise While Losing Weight?

As you progress through your weight loss struggle, you can expect a boost to your confidence and self-esteem. Depending upon your mental stability, it is likely that you will start opening yourself up to a lot of new opportunities, especially socialisation. However, one of the biggest problems I faced when it came to socialising was the eating aspect. I was always concerned about eating the wrong food and concomitantly falling into a relapse. I was very frightened of submitting to a moment of weakness by overeating thereby undoing all my previous achievements. I always tried to avoid social gatherings such as family union, religious celebrations, evening dinners and birthday parties, all of which I regarded as "danger zones". As all these events had one thing in common — lots of food to eat and plenty of liquor to drink — there was a great danger of vulnerability to a relapse during or straight after the completion of these events. This was an area where I showed my greatest weakness. Avoiding all social events would have solved this problem, but I did not want to miss out on opportunities which I could exploit to build on my social skills and network with other people. As a result, I had to make a few adjustments here and there to accommodate social events and also getting engaged in other weight loss activities.

Below are some of the strategies I had employed during socialisation:

+ I filled my stomach before I participated in events. This ensured that I did not give myself an opportunity to pig out later;

+ I stopped using social situations to have a "cheat day"; I made sure that I stayed true to my clean diet;

+ If I took something at social events, I ensured that I did not consume alcohol or eat any sugary food;

+ I left all my money and bank cards at home; this ensured that I would not buy junk food on the way home;

+ I ensured that I had no sugary foods at home to devour after attending social events; and

+ I got into the habit of saying 'No' when faced with peer pressure at social events to take alcohol and eat superfluously.

Socialising has been a big issue for me since I started my weight loss efforts. I have had situations where a bad night out, or just eating one wrong food, had triggered a relapse and unraveled months of progressive work. Such experiences subsequently made me avoid all types of socialising that involved eating or drinking. However, the tips I have given above had immensely helped me to find a balance between losing weight and socialisation.

My Weight Loss Efforts are Getting Slower

Losing weight by exercising and dieting is a very slow process, and it is something that you will have to embrace and entertain. You should know by now that after successfully completing your exercising and dieting routines you should expect some permanent changes to your lifestyle. Remember there is no easy way to lose body weight, and you will have to do all the hard work over a reasonable period of time. For example, if you have been living in an unhealthy lifestyle for twenty years, you cannot possibly expect to reverse your sorry state of affairs in twenty days, or even three months. Not only will you have to give your body adequate time for changes to manifest themselves, but it would also be unreasonable for you to expect that you can undo years of damage in a few weeks.

Assuming that you have a solid weight loss strategy in place and are able to get through your exercises on a daily basis, you should initially expect fat to burn off easily. Consider this beginner's luck. However, it is important to remember that this initial rapid weight loss is not permanent, and once this phase is over the rate of fat you burn will begin to slow down. It will then take you to spend more time and effort to accelerate the fat-burning process. It is important for you to remember this information so that you do not display extreme smugness and laxity at the initial stage and then regret later for any untoward consequences.

During my weight struggle, I burnt with ease a lot of fat at the initial stage. I was overjoyed when I found out that I had lost approximately a kilogram a week. However, one of the serious mistakes I had made at this stage was my expectation that I would continue to lose weight at this rate right throughout my Journey. This did not happen because a number of changes took place during the passage of time, which either accelerated or impeded my progress. So, initially I lost weight, but this slowed down afterwards. As I had not lost much weight at the beginning of my Journey, I felt demoralised and expressed doubt about the efficacy of my programme. I felt as if I had not organised my dieting properly, or that I was not exercising enough. Obviously, I needed a different approach because, as the diagram on the Point of No Return shows, some stages in the Journey will be more difficult to plough through than others. This is so because it takes more time and effort to burn fat during difficult stages. So, if your progress has slowed during the difficult stages, it should not in any way be interpreted as a reflection of your inadequacy. Don't be dejected and don't let doubt dwell upon you, continue to eat clean and exercise. Yes, you may have to make changes to your diet and exercise patterns, but give your weight loss plan adequate time to work.

Feeling Unhappy

There is a misconception that eating healthy food and exercising regularly should give us the feeling of happiness every single minute of our lives. Ideally, every morning we should see ourselves jumping straight out of bed and ready to take on the world. In fact, you will be disappointed when you realise that this has not happened, as you will continue to face days when you still need to drag yourself out of bed and go through a below-average day despite all the progress you have made. For example, extraneous influences such as sick and elderly parents, bad weather, job pressures, mortgage stress and family problems, inter alia, will continue to greatly impact on your progress and life. They will not magically disappear from your life as the result of your efforts. It is expected that these factors would make us feel sad over a long period of time. Thus, no amount of eating healthy food and exercising will dispel these extraneous influences. However, the endorphins that is introduced into the body from exercising is an excellent agent in changing negative thought patterns and improving your mood. However, they alone will not lead you to a state of permanent bliss nor suppress any unpleasant emotion.

When we see our favourite health celebrities showing us how awesome their lives are because of their healthy living, remember that we do not get an accurate portrayal of their life, but a glimpse of them doing their job. They are paid to sell us happiness and promote a lifestyle which should make us feel awesome and self-fulfilled. Do not be fooled.

I want you to appreciate all the emotions that you go through every day and understand that they are there for a reason. It is a part of life. Also, do understand that no amount of healthy eating and exercising will give you permanent happiness. You will still have your good and bad days. Even the healthiest and wealthiest people we know don't wake up every day feeling awesome and happy, and, like you, also experience periods of life without happiness. So, enjoy your good days and continue to work on minimising the bad ones.

Do Not Compare Yourself to Other People

We all have a tendency to compare ourselves to others. Whether it be at school, work, sports or how we look, it is a very bad habit that has been drilled into us from a very young age. Even to this day, I still compare myself to others, especially on weight loss progress, building muscles and physical appearance. If I ever see a person who is taller, better looking or muscular than me, I automatically start feeling inferior to him, and wish I had possessed their traits and attractive physical features. However, you must remember that comparing yourself to other people is demoralising and inane. It serves no other purpose than to rob you of your happiness and time. Every time I compare myself to other people, I always end up judging myself harshly and feeling inferior. This is because the people who supply the information, especially on weight loss and muscle building activities, invariably exaggerate their results. I had found that there were a few people who had claimed that they had:

+ Successfully deadlifted 200 kilograms in their first attempt;
+ Lost 20 kilos in 4 weeks;
+ Put on 10 kilos of muscle in 2 weeks; and
+ Achieved their physique naturally when they actually took a ton of supplements.

So, what we see or hear from others may not actually be true. There is always the possibility that the persons who make you feel bad and inferior may lack legitimacy. Such people could just be bullshit artists who try to inflate their egos. I have no doubt that you will be setting yourself for failure if you compare your progress with others. Thus, the best action you should take is to compare yourself to your former self. This is what I did. By choosing this option I got motivated to be my best self. However, if you do have to compare yourself with another person, you should look for their strengths as a learning tool. In this way, you could mimic their work ethic and obtain inspiration from their Journey.

Next time you happen to compare yourself with another person, ask yourself several times if you would also trade places with them. You cannot just cherry pick. Would you be happy to take on all their problems and sufferings along with all the good qualities they have?

CHAPTER 3

Maintenance: Remaining slim after Losing Weight

Once you have successfully completed your Journey and successfully achieved your goals and objectives, then it is time to shift your gear into the maintenance mode. This is the last stage in your struggle where you will have to sustain the results that you have achieved. If you are under the impression that your Journey is over now, then you are abysmally wrong. This is so because you will still need to continue monitoring and maintaining the results of your changed lifestyle, in order to enjoy the results on a long-term basis, and to ensure that you do not return to your former self.

As mentioned in the previous chapters, it is very easy to undo all the hard work that you have put in to complete your Journey. It is for this reason that you must be very vigilant and find time to sustain your gains.

As part of my maintenance plan, I have implemented a long-term strategy to maintain my new lifestyle. This includes continuation of exercising on a regular basis, playing gamification, and permanent adoption of a healthier, sugar free diet. Even though I am occasionally tempted to binge out on junk food, I try my best to totally avoid this temptation. I know from previous experience how one moment of weakness can easily trigger off a relapse. On a number of occasions during my Journey I had experienced loss of efforts and achievements apparently due to deviation from my established weight-loss plan, and I have learnt from my mistakes.

That is why I ensure that even though I have accomplished my weight-loss goals, I still refrain from engaging in activities that will take me back to my old eating habits and lifestyle.

The gamification elements that I have added to my maintenance plan have underpinned my ability to further sustain my changed lifestyle and physical transformation. By playing gamification, I am continually working with my strengths and have been able to set more interesting and challenging goals for accomplishment. Some of my future challenges include going without alcohol for a whole year and soft drinks for three years. By setting such goals, I am ensuring that I do not feel as if my Journey has ended or that there is nothing else left for me to achieve thus leaving me complacent and lonely.

I must also point out that I have made a number of mistakes at this stage of my struggle and, based on my experience, I have this important advice for you: Do not be fooled into thinking that you can always return to your old eating habits once you have overcome obesity, because you will find it very difficult to reverse any tendency towards recidivism. In other words, do you want to go back to your former self? Please do not underestimate how fast you can go into a relapse and how fast you can put back all your weight without realisation. So, the best way to sustain change is to completely sacrifice your old lifestyle. This is the only way to achieve permanent results.

You must also ensure that you continue ways to improve your life in other areas. You can now push yourself even further as you are no longer limited by your weight. Put all your energy towards self-actualisation - Master Yourself.

At the end of the day, remember that it is a huge achievement for you to have reached this stage. You have now achieved your weight loss dream. Ensure that you do all you can to avoid a recrudescence of your former self.

Changing Your Mentality

I have read somewhere that our "bodies may change, but the mind stays the same." So, once you have achieved your weight loss objectives, you may find yourself adjusting to your new life psychologically challenging. If you have been overweight for a significant period, you will find that your mind has become used to a certain way of thinking. While the conclusion of your struggle will have a positive impact on your mentality, it will not completely heal it. For example, despite the fact I have achieved my weight loss goals, I continue to see myself as an overweight individual. There are numerous occasions where I allowed my 'imaginary' weight to hold me back from enjoying my new life-style despite the fact that I am not overweight anymore. I realised this phenomenon as a problem while out shopping some time ago when I had entered a store and asked the shop assistant for a shirt sized 3XL. The sales lady started laughing and told me that the shirt size was too big for me. I had completely forgotten that I was not that overweight person anymore, yet I continued to think like my former self. The point I am trying to make here is that even though I have changed physically, I feel I am still the same person mentally. Despite my physical transformation, I still believe that no women will ever show romantic interest in me, or the ladder will break if I step on it, or a person will not be able to lift me up if I fainted on the street. So, I have yet to adjust mentally to my new self. If you encounter this issue after your endeavour, then you must sit down and regularly remind yourself that you are not the same person anymore. If people still treat you as if nothing has changed, accept this unreality and act accordingly. If you get invited to parties, accept the invitation and go out. If a girl shows interest, make a move with alacrity. You must open yourself and accept the rewards you have reaped.

Don't hold back, as it will prevent you from accepting your new life and all the opportunities that have come with it.

If you continue to live with your old mind in a new body, you will never experience the full potential of what you have achieved. Your Journey will still be incomplete. So, while working on your physical self, also take the time to reinvigorate your mental faculty as well, and start living your new life with a brand-new set of lenses.

You Deserve Happiness

Once you have successfully lost weight, and depending on how much weight you have lost, you will find that you will need to undertake surgery to address problems related to excess skin. This can be major or minor surgery, depending on how much excess skin there is for removal. This medical intervention will be a frustrating experience for you, given the tremendous amount of time and efforts you had spent in achieving your weight loss goals.

If you face the issue of excessive skin on your tummy after dieting, current cosmetic surgery is available to correct this baggage. Body contouring after massive weight loss procedures can be undertaken to eliminate excess skin once a significant amount of weight has been lost. Regretfully, several operations may be required to fully address your concerns. These procedures need to be planned over the course of months, and even years. However, as medical technology is continually changing, it would be best to discuss treatment options with your doctor and medical specialists regarding the best treatment. Do note that it is best to only consider this path once your weight has been stable for 6 to 12 months after completing your Journey.

Relapse

During your Journey, you may find yourself in a situation when you do not feel confident enough to continue with your weight loss initiatives despite trying your best to stick to your routine. This may eventually lead you to give up the current struggle and consequently reverting to your previous unhealthy lifestyle. This occurrence is known as a relapse.

During my struggle, I had experienced a relapse on many occasions. Unfortunately, this event is one of the most disappointing, self-conscious and painful experiences that I have endured. Not only does it have the potential to undo all the hard work that you have already put together to change your lifestyle, but it also has the potential to take you back to your original self, or even to a state worse than that.

There is a variety of reasons why a person can fall into a relapse. These reasons include unrealistic expectations, extreme methods for quick weight loss, stress, death in a family, people or places that are linked to your unhealthy lifestyle, emotional issues, reminders of your unhealthy lifestyle in the media (e.g advertisements), family gathering and festive seasons and, my personal favourite, a "cheat day" gone wrong. It is vital to remember that these issues, inter alia, no matter how large or small, can trigger a relapse. So, it is vital that you have preventative measures in place to minimise the possibility of the occurrence of this situation. You must also ensure that once you have relapsed you do not discontinue your entire Journey. Do not let a relapse affect your progress or momentum. Accept that a relapse has happened, and slowly start rebuilding your momentum. You can do this by slowly transitioning back to your healthy lifestyle. Reduce your exercise load for a few days, do the minimum if you have to, and then slowly build up speed. Initially, if you have to force yourself to get back on track, do so. During my Journey, I found that sometimes force was the only way to get restarted and that it is something one will have to get used to. However, you will find that the first 2-3 days are a real struggle, but usually after 5 to 6 days you will be back on track feeling as if you had never gone through a relapse.

Going through a relapse is part and parcel of the weight loss struggle. You will encounter it at one point or the other. However, one of the most important things to remember during a relapse is that you should not beat yourself up or feel that you have completely blown up your entire progress. Do not feel as if you have somehow failed. Becoming and remaining healthy is a life-long process and there will be humps along the way. However, you must always pick yourself up and continue walking towards your targeted goal.

Don't give a relapse time to grow. It will be very easy to tell yourself that this is just a one-off event and that you will try to avoid it the next time. This is procrastination. This is not good enough, for soon you will find yourself moving in a downward spiral. You have to give the highest priority to the treatment of a relapse.

Some strategies that I had used in dealing with and bouncing back from a relapse included:

+ Take personal responsibility for the situation and immediately work on getting back on track;
+ Make a note of the warning signs of a potential relapse, and identifying ways to solve the problem;
+ Use relapse as a positive experience to reassess my weight loss plan, and make the appropriate changes;
+ Ensure that I maintain a positive attitude throughout the entire ordeal;

- Use the assistance of friends and family to get back on track;
- Spend time watching health videos and browsing bodybuilding fora to build motivation;
- Use gamification techniques, which I discussed earlier in this book, to re-kick-start my weight loss plan;
- Use force and willpower to get back on track, if required; and
- Understand that just because I had a relapse does not mean that I have returned instantly to my original self.

By adopting and utilising the above techniques, I have ensured that I have a procedure in place to address a large number of issues related to a relapse.

The Importance of Remembering

We tend to forget how we felt during times when we were overweight.

- Very easy to forget.
- Make sure you do not forget.

Achieving Success

Any successful weight loss journey will entail a lot of time, effort and hard work. Your Journey will be no different. Based on my experience, the final success or achievement can be described as an iceberg as shown in Figure 6 on p129. As this diagram shows, people around you will only see your success but they will rarely experience the frustrations and hurdles that lie underneath the iceberg.

During my Journey, I noticed that almost all my friends and

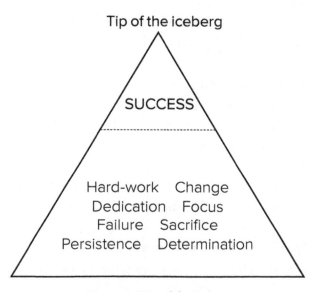

Tip of the iceberg

SUCCESS

Hard-work   Change
Dedication   Focus
Failure   Sacrifice
Persistence   Determination

Figure 6: Tip of the Iceberg

family members failed to realise how much hard work I had devoted to my weight loss programme. They assumed that there was some magic behind my success. However, this was not the case. The bottom section, under SUCCESS, in the iceberg aptly applies to my struggle. Let me explain my failures in particular. I had failed so many times while trying to lose weight. I had tried and tried, but success still eluded me. People in my circle never saw me as a person who tried and failed but as somebody who deliberately accumulated weight. I was profoundly disappointed at my repeated failures and reversion to my original shape — disappointed that so much time and effort had gone to waste; disappointed because I felt that I just didn't have the ingredients needed to succeed; disappointed because I could see my life ebbing away at the most critical stage of my life. I became severely depressed and hated myself even more as I saw myself as a person who lacked self-control and body discipline. My family and friends never tried to understand my disappointments. I sacrificed a lot to succeed, especially by rigorous dieting. I ended up giving up all sugary and junk food and took a higher intake of fruits and vegetables. I cleaned my life by adopting a minimalistic lifestyle. During freezing winter months, I forced myself to wake up early in the morning for exercising. My final success would not have been possible without these herculean efforts and struggles, which people never experienced nor recognised. I understand many people do not change even when faced with adversities, but I did. I really wanted to change my body and I was prepared to adopt the tactics and strategies to achieve my weighty objectives. Opening my mind to different lifestyles, unconventional knowledge and ideas enabled me to achieve a new lifestyle.

Conclusion and Moving Forward

Obesity is one of the fastest growth 'diseases' in the world. Scientists and pharmaceutical companies still have not been able to come out with a total cure for this problem. What we do acknowledge is that a simple weighty problem can easily be conquered or mitigated by a person with a show of determination, courage and dedication. But genetic-based obesity is a bit difficult to attack because it will involve severe dieting, exercising and surgery. Very obese people can also reduce their body weight, but not by dieting alone. They will need surgery for the removal of loose skin. Now that I have successfully completed my Journey, my future will be preoccupied with the maintenance of my new body. My entire journey has been an incredible experience, one that has taught me the value of self-discipline, persistence, and dedication. It has also revealed my true personality. This experience enabled me to become the person I have always envisioned to be. The success that I have experienced has also made me believe that each and every one of us have the ability to lose weight and live the life of choice — a life without barriers. That is why I am confident that you will complete your Journey.

Before I let you go, I want you to know that I may not know you personally and most likely will never meet you, but if you are currently suffering from obesity or other weight related issues, I want you to know that I can better relate to your struggle and that nothing would make me happier than to see you overcome it. I thank you for taking time to read my book and I convey my best wishes during your Journey.

CHECKLIST

STRATEGIES TO GUIDE YOU THROUGH EACH STAGE OF YOUR JOURNEY

STAGE	STRATEGIES
Pre-contemplation	
Contemplation	
Preparation	
Action	
Maintenance	
Action	

REFERENCES

1. Fat, Sick and Nearly Dead (Film). Viewed in *https://www.youtube.com/User/FatSickandNearlyDead* on 25th December 2016.

2. Government of Newfoundland and Labrador (2005). Strategic Planning Facilitator Guide. Viewed in *http://www.ibrd.gov.nl.ca/regionaldev/ccb/stratplan/ccb_stratplan-facilitatorguide.pdf* on 5th February 2017.

3. Leeder, S. (2017) Obesity crisis can't be ignored. Let's start talking before it's too late. *Sunday Telegraph*, 15th January, pp. 36-37.

4. Lustig, R. H. Sugar-The Bitter Truth (Video) Viewed in *http://www.uctv.tv/Shows/Sugar-The-Bitter-Truth-16717*, 16th January 2016.

5. Martin, P. (2017). A new year diet that might actually work. Sunday *The Sun-Herald*, 1st January, 2017, p.30.

6. Oz, Dr. Cheat on Your Diet and still lose weight. The Dr. Oz show. Viewed in *http://www.doctoroz.com/print/44349* on 13th December 2016.

7. Peel, C. (2017). Fat Kids a $17m health burden. *Daily Telegraph*, 24th January, p. 3.

8. Prochaska, J.O, C C. DiClemente and J. C. Norcross (1992). In Search of How People Change. Applications to Addictive Behavior. *American Psychologist*, 47(9), 1102-1114.

9. Robbins, A. (2001). *Awake the giant within. How to Take Immediate Control of your Mental, Emotional, Physical and Financial Destiny!* Pocket Books, London, p. 24.

10. Robbins, A. (2001). *op.cit.* p.26.

11. Robbins, A. (2001): *op. cit*, p. 26-27.
12. Robbins, A. (2001). *op.cit*, pp. 316-317
13. Robbins, A. (2001). *op.cit*, pp 440-41.